Singapore's First Year of COVID-19

Kenneth Paul Tan
Editor

Singapore's First Year of COVID-19

Public Health, Immigration, the Neoliberal State,
and Authoritarian Populism

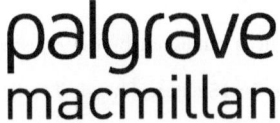

Editor
Kenneth Paul Tan
School of Communication and Film
Hong Kong Baptist University
Kowloon Tong, Hong Kong

ISBN 978-981-19-0367-0   ISBN 978-981-19-0368-7   (eBook)
https://doi.org/10.1007/978-981-19-0368-7

Cover illustration: © Melisa Hasan

This Palgrave Macmillan imprint is published by the registered company Springer Nature Singapore Pte Ltd.
The registered company address is: 152 Beach Road, #21-01/04 Gateway East, Singapore 189721, Singapore

Acknowledgements

This book began as a new research-intensive course that I had designed for a group of nine double-degree Masters students, who were going to spend the second year of their studies at the National University of Singapore's (NUS) Lee Kuan Yew School of Public Policy (LKY School), after completing their first year at Sciences Po in Paris. Having worked at NUS for a little over two decades, this was also going to be my final year as a professor at the LKY School, before taking up a new position as a Professor of Politics, Film, and Cultural Studies at Hong Kong Baptist University. As an academic with interdisciplinary interests and one who had always been excited about finding synergies among teaching, research, and service, I wanted to finish with a bang.

And so I designed a course that would take students through the process of collaboratively writing a book, under my supervision, with the rather brazen aim of getting it published. Its subject would be Singapore's experience of the COVID-19 pandemic that, when the course began in August 2020, had already made its presence profoundly felt in the global city for more than half a year. This was a "live" case that I wanted the students to use as a kind of "x-ray" lens for seeing through the full regalia of one of the wealthiest countries in the world, to see Singapore in its full naked glory, warts and all.

But most of these students who were from Europe, North America, and China had never been to Singapore before. I needed to provide them with a "starter kit" of Singapore studies literature, which has grown tremendously over the last couple of decades, and a theoretical framework that would unify the research, or at least make it coherent enough for an edited volume. So we read and discussed as much of that literature as we could, and the students also enrolled in another Singapore-focused course that I was teaching that semester called "Pragmatism and Public Morality in Singapore" (or "Sex, Drugs, and Rock & Roll", as we affectionately called it). As for a theoretical framework, we engaged with some ideas that I had been working on more generally, ideas that were associated with neoliberal globalization, authoritarian populism, and moral panic. I outlined the chapters of the book in the broadest terms and asked students to choose which they were interested to write. From these starting points, the students went off to conduct independent research and draft their chapters collaboratively. We met as a class very regularly, mostly through Zoom. The students presented their drafts and received detailed constructive criticism from me and their fellow students.

A vital part of the process involved interacting with a few activists and experts on the subject. I invited them individually for long Zoom meetings at which they spoke about their experiences and answered our many questions. This book has without a doubt benefitted greatly from the wisdom, passion, and generosity of Alex Au, Cai Yinzhou, Debbie Fordyce, Jeremy Lim, Ong Suan Ee, Jolovan Wham, and Joanne Yoong. We also benefitted from administrative assistance provided by the always awesome Academic Affairs team at the LKY School, including Lela Mohamed, Florence Siew, and Agnes Tan. Vishal Daryanomel, a Senior Commissioning Editor at Palgrave Macmillan, was enormously encouraging and incredibly efficient in taking the process forward, which included obtaining very helpful reports from three anonymous reviewers. To everyone mentioned here, the authors of this book are extremely grateful.

And finally, I would like to thank my students for working with me on this book project. The amount of effort and commitment that have gone into it far exceed what normal coursework would demand. I am very proud of you all.

Hong Kong   Kenneth Paul Tan
October 2021

CONTENTS

Contents

Editor and Contributors

About the Editor

Kenneth Paul Tan is Professor of Politics, Film, and Cultural Studies, School of Communication and Film, Hong Kong Baptist University; formerly Associate Professor, Lee Kuan Yew School of Public Policy, National University of Singapore.

Chapter authors were his students who graduated in 2021 with a Double Master Degree in Public Policy and European Affairs from the National University of Singapore and Sciences Po.

List of Contributors

Carolin Bernhard Neustadt, Germany

Davide Brugola Carbonate, Italy

Johanna Dirlewanger-Lücke Brussels, Belgium

Andrea Dugo Corsico, Italy

Mara Ellemunt Perca, Italy

Michael Flood Paris, France

Junhao Li Shenzhen, China

Hongwu Lyu Hangzhou, China

Aymeric Vo Quang Versailles, France

LIST OF TABLES

CHAPTER 1

Neoliberal Globalization, Authoritarian Populism, and Moral Panics

Kenneth Paul Tan

Abstract At the start of Singapore's first year of living with COVID-19, its government was praised internationally for its ability to control the spread of the virus through high standards of testing, tracing, and isolation, the basic elements of communicable disease control. Its success strengthened both its brand as a global city and its national narrative often referred to as "The Singapore Story". However, the first year of COVID-19 also exposed weaknesses in the Singapore system of development, governance, and policymaking. And yet, that very same system seemed, at least on the surface, sufficiently resilient to correct the immediate problems and adapt to changing circumstances. The question perhaps is whether the Singapore system is capable of further adapting in the face of intensifying volatility, uncertainly, complexity, and ambiguity, the kind of future of which COVID-19 might in fact be merely a portent. How should lapses such as the serious outbreak of infection in the migrant

K. P. Tan (✉)
School of Communication and Film, Hong Kong Baptist University, Kowloon Tong, Hong Kong
e-mail: kennethptan@hkbu.edu.hk

© The Author(s), under exclusive license to Springer Nature Singapore Pte Ltd. 2022
K. P. Tan (ed.), *Singapore's First Year of COVID-19*,
https://doi.org/10.1007/978-981-19-0368-7_1

worker dormitories be viewed? It is reasonable to admit that no government is perfect, not even in well-governed Singapore. One can also say that crisis of this kind can be unpredictable and so all one can hope for is that the authorities did the best that they could, given what they knew and the resources that they possessed. But, from these lapses, one could also gain insight into deeper problems of a structural or systemic nature. Putting out the proverbial fires, difficult as it is to do, may distract from their real causes, which could be subterranean, or climatic, or ideological. These causes are deeper than a simple explanatory chain linking events, behaviour, decisions, responsibility, and corrections. These deeper causes are all linked in some way to neoliberal globalization and authoritarian populist responses to it.

Keywords The Singapore Story · The Singapore brand · Neoliberal globalization · Authoritarian populism · Moral panic · VUCA world · Resilience

PANDEMIC IN SINGAPORE: YEAR ONE

By 11 March 2021, exactly one year after the World Health Organization (WHO) had declared COVID-19 a global pandemic, the virus had infected over 118 million people, claiming 2.6 million lives worldwide (Heng and Au, 2021).

Beyond these very concerning numbers and their epidemiological context, the pandemic had already provoked transformations in nearly every domain of human life, including the economic, social, cultural, psychological, technological, ecological, political, geopolitical, and their various intersections, at levels that ranged from the local to the global. In most instances, the pandemic had forcefully accelerated trends that were already recognized years earlier in future-oriented thinking. Work-from-home, home-based learning, and online deliveries, so much now a part of daily life even in the first year of COVID-19, had already been anticipated in the "future of work", "future of education", and "future of business" discussion themes both framing and shaping the common imagination of future scenarios in preparation for the threats and opportunities presented by the disruptions of the "fourth industrial revolution" (Schwab, 2015).

Many of these pre-COVID-19 discussions about the future had recognized that disruption would create benefits and costs whose distribution would be anything but even. Some would benefit more than others. And some would pay a much higher price than others. The COVID-19 pandemic brought about an economic downturn at all levels, which was expected to be painfully protracted, though its effects were not equally felt among richer and poorer countries, and within countries where the more advantaged were naturally better able to cope and perhaps even to profit by it. Vaccines, whose development had been urgently expedited, were being rolled out, though poorer and less powerful countries and communities had significantly less access to them, at least initially. Variants of the virus, which appeared especially in places with poor access to vaccines and public health facilities, began to reinfect even the well-vaccinated countries and communities as they gradually opened, thus dampening hopes of rapidly attaining herd immunity (UN News, 2021). Meanwhile, ideology, politics, conspiratorial thinking, and misinformation, spread efficiently and rapidly through social media and messaging networks, fuelled vaccine hesitancy and resistance to public health measures such as mask-wearing and safe distancing (Roozenbeek et al., 2020).

Determined to keep their economies afloat, the more courageous governments—criticized from other perspectives as foolhardy—worked together on establishing travel bubbles that would enable people movement between partner countries without the paralyzing need for quarantine (Chew, 2021). Among these more proactively globalist governments, eager to convey the message that they are always open for business, has been the government of Singapore (Toh, 2020).

This book aims to document critically the first year of COVID-19 in Singapore. It focuses specifically on the interconnections among Singapore's political economy, public health policies, immigration policies, and the elite and pragmatic system of state authoritarianism that, especially since the 1980s, has been at the heart of managing the tensions and contradictions of a nation-state that is also a global city (Tan, 2017).

In January 2020, at the start of Singapore's first year of living with COVID-19, its government was praised internationally for its ability to control the spread of the virus through high standards of testing, tracing, and isolation, the basic elements of communicable disease control ("WHO praises Singapore's response to coronavirus outbreak", 2020). And quite remarkably, Singapore was able to achieve this even though, as a global city of the first rank, its boundaries were among the most porous in the world. Its success has strengthened both its brand as a global city and its national narrative often referred to as "The Singapore Story". The Singapore brand is a carefully managed projection of an external image to boost Singapore's attractiveness and appeal for economic and diplomatic purposes. An effective national brand can help to amplify Singapore's international influence that is always limited by its diminutive size.

The Singapore Story is an internally directed over-arching account of what it has taken for Singapore to survive and prosper, in the context of structural challenges and opportunities. This official narrative serves as reference points to unify and inspire the people of Singapore, to orientate policy choices, to provide reasons to justify ideological positions and political actions, and ultimately to help legitimize and gain broad acceptance of the authoritarian regime. At the centre of this regime is the People's Action Party (PAP) that has been in power since 1959. Therefore, while the national narrative provides content to the Singapore identity and legitimizes the state's monopoly and extensive use of domestic power, the global-city brand augments its limited external influence with "soft power" (Tan, K.P., 2018). Singapore's initially successful pandemic response boosted both narrative and brand.

And then, within just a few months, that glowing reputation tarnished rapidly. Infection rates suddenly began to rise significantly among migrant workers who were housed in gated dormitories. Their poor living conditions contrasted shamefully—or worse, shamelessly—with the glistening first-world global city, which migrant workers had built and cleaned for decades. The situation was reported in several major news outlets around the world, many criticizing not so much Singapore's handling of the outbreak, but its policies towards and treatment of migrant workers, some of the most vulnerable people living and working in the country. These news reports included "Packed with migrant workers, dormitories fuel Coronavirus in Singapore" in *The New York Times* (Cai and Lai, 2020), "Singapore was a Coronavirus success story—Until an outbreak showed how vulnerable workers can fall through the cracks" in *Time* (Leung, 2020), and "Singapore's cramped migrant worker dorms hide Covid-19 surge risk" in *The Guardian* (Ratcliffe, 2020). From Singapore's moral blind spot emerged the country's most serious COVID-19 clusters, drawing international attention to structural weaknesses in the system. It took several months to bring the situation under control. And yet, a year-and-a-half later, the workers, who had by that time nearly all been vaccinated, were still practically imprisoned within these dorms, confronted by mental health issues including suicide. Articles such as "Singapore's migrant workers have endured interminable lockdowns" in *The Economist* (2021) and "In lockdown for 18 months, Singapore's migrant workers yearn for freedom" in *The New York Times* (Young, 2021) continue to direct international attention to a problem that seems determined to stay in the country's moral blind spot, increasingly overshadowed by political rather than public health considerations.

This book does not attempt to assess Singapore's overall performance in the first year of COVID-19 and to compare it with that of others such as Taiwan, South Korea, and New Zealand, greatly admired internationally for their consistently successful management of the pandemic (Glasgow, 2020). Indeed, such a comparative assessment would be quite futile, given the bewildering array of factors, unintended consequences, and still evolving outcomes associated with something as complex and rapidly unfurling as this pandemic. The uncertainty of a post-pandemic future—given how challenging it is at the time of writing this book to even imagine when the pandemic will end—should warn us against the hubris of so hastily proclaiming success or failure, even as leaders attempt to draw lessons from an expanding well of collective experience for dealing with more immediate problems.

Instead, the chapters in this book recognize how the first year of COVID-19 has sufficiently exposed weaknesses in the Singapore system of development, governance, and policymaking, so often vaunted by leaders of all stripes around the world. And yet, that very same system seemed, at least on the surface, sufficiently resilient to correct the immediate problems and adapt to changing circumstances. The question perhaps is whether the Singapore system is capable of further adapting in the face of intensifying volatility, uncertainly, complexity, and ambiguity, the kind of future of which COVID-19 might in fact be merely a portent.

How should lapses such as the serious dormitory clusters be viewed? It is reasonable to admit that no government is perfect, not even in well-governed Singapore. One can also say that crisis of this kind can be unpredictable and so all one can hope for is that the authorities did the best that they could, given what they knew and the resources that they possessed. But, from these lapses, one could also gain insight into deeper problems of a structural or systemic nature. Putting out the proverbial fires, difficult as it is to do, may distract from their real causes, which could be subterranean, or climatic, or ideological. The chapters in this book aim to identify causes that are deeper than a simple explanatory chain linking events, behaviour, decisions, responsibility, and corrections. These deeper causes, the book suggests, are all linked in some way to neoliberal globalization and authoritarian populist responses to it.

Becoming a Neoliberal Global City

S. Rajaratnam was a prominent member of independent Singapore's founding generation of political leaders. His description in a 1972 speech of Singapore as a "global city" is often cited and celebrated for its prescience. The term, in its highly influential contemporary sense (Sassen, 1991), had yet to be academically formalized and widely used in scholarly or even policy circles, but it captured the essence of how Singapore was and continues to be understood as a small and vulnerable state with limited natural resources. As such, its connectedness with the rest of the world not only presented opportunities for flourishing—amidst many economic, political, social, and cultural risks—but also established the very basis upon which Singapore could survive. Thus, in many ways, the language of the global city has been, since Singapore's earliest decades of independence, a fundamental and vital ideational resource for constructing Singapore's self-knowledge, existential realization, and even external brand image (Tan, K.P., 2018).

However, it was really only since the mid-1980s that global-city Singapore transformed into a qualitatively new entity, what I shall call the neoliberal global city. This new entity, I argue, can best be made sense of through the lens of neoliberal globalization, a theoretical framework that exposes and critiques the excesses of extreme capitalism that all over the world pervades, devalues, and degrades local identities and capacities for democracy, social justice, moral solidarity, and human security. In their place, one finds instead synthetic, top-down, and pious assertions of national unity, loyalty, and security threats often fabricated, or simply exaggerated, to serve the interests of the powerful and wealthy (Harvey, 2005; Giroux, 2004; Scholte, 2005).

Neoliberalism itself begins quite innocuously, suggesting from its own name a renewed, perhaps improved, primacy given to freedom, which is at the heart of classical liberalism. Freedom here refers to individual freedom as the basis of social good, as it did in classical liberalism. But with neoliberalism, individual freedom is achieved almost exclusively through the market. Not just the myriad individual transactions that are mediated and coordinated through the mechanisms and dynamics of the market, but also the very logic of the market that in its pervasive and expansive nature is thought to maximize individual freedom. In reality, this market logic debases the social, moral, aesthetic, and other domains of the lifeworld (Sandel, 2012). One manifestation of the primacy of the market is the way in which hyper-competitiveness atomizes people, making them feel precarious in all respects, constraining any possibility of moral solidarity, and restricting the sense of responsibility that one might have for others in their community.

The state's role, according to neoliberalism, is not to roll back and make way for the market to take over, but to protect and enhance the market, whose mechanisms, dynamics, and logics enable individual freedom and therefore the social good to be maximized. The state, in actuality, fortifies itself to protect property rights against the power of labour and social movements. Its role, in a sense, is to protect those who have (more) property from those who do not (have as much). Its language, cloaked in seemingly neutral technocratic pragmatism, disguises what really amounts to market fundamentalism. A regressive role like this requires the strength and resolve of an authoritarian state, one that wields repressive instruments such as the civil administration, the police, the courts, and the prisons, as well as ideological instruments to shape and control the common-sense thinking, speech, and actions of its citizens to produce and maintain consensus on neoliberal globalization as the only game in town that one has no choice but play to win.

The neoliberal-authoritarian state aligns itself with corporate power, forming an elite partnership between state and corporate capital. The neoliberal elite is constituted through this union, which is not always frictionless. The elite disguise their interests through a rhetoric of technocratic pragmatism, which claims that the government makes decisions that are free of ideological and moralistic dogma, focuses on the achievement of results through the implementation of the most efficient, effective, and impactful techniques; borrows ideas that it likes from anywhere to adapt intelligently to the local context; and accepts the immutability of real-world constraints, preferring to work realistically around them rather than to attempt idealistically to transform them (Tan, 2017).

Paradoxically, this anti-ideological mode of pragmatism conceals a deeper ideology: neoliberal globalization. When the results being focused upon are tethered to efficiency and economic growth, especially as they benefit the elite, Singapore-style technocracy can hardly be ideologically

neutral, even as it strains to disseminate a belief in the trickle-down benefits for everyone of looking after the rich and powerful. Technocracy itself
assumes a highly managerial style of government that not only devalues
the significance of politics and broader social participation for governance,
but also careerizes public service to an extreme level while replacing
leadership with managerial bureaucracy. The New Public Management
movement, though "revolutionary" in the 1990s for shaking up the
dysfunctionality of public service everywhere in the world by subjecting
it to the exacting logic of consumerism, continues into the Singapore of
the present as policy inertia, held back by conservative and unimagina-
tive budgets and bottom lines, deferential organizational hierarchies, and
self-preserving groupthink.

Perversely, in order to maximize individual freedom the neoliberal way,
the state has had to roll not back—as classical liberals might have argued—
but out even further and often in more nuanced and sophisticated
ways to exercise a higher degree of social control. Economic freedom,
in this view, necessitates authoritarian control—two sides of the same
coin—chiefly to tame and productively harness the energies of society in
order to advance first and foremost the interests of the capitalist elite.
This has meant corporatizing the unions, atomizing the workforce into
hyper-competitive and even precarious rivals, and thus "depoliticizing"
the labour movement so that wages, benefits, and work conditions can
be determined technocratically and demands for improvement neutered
through institutionalized control.

Thus, it is hardly surprising to learn that Singapore ranks very highly
among cities with overworked people, and very poorly when it comes
to work-life balance (Kisi, 2020). Work-oriented Singaporeans are among
the most sleep-deprived in the world (Tan, S.Y., 2018). A World Health
Organization report using 2015 data showed Singapore to have the
highest rate of depression in Asia. Singapore is consistently ranked among
the most expensive cities in the world (Economist Intelligence Unit,
2020). Income inequality, as measured by the Gini index, is well above
the OECD average and points to the possibility of social unrest (Smith
et al., 2015).

The gleaming global city, whose reputation for rapid development,
strong governance, and innovative policymaking has been admired by so
many, is—upon closer inspection—also a highly unequal, individualistic,
demoralizing, repressed, and cynical society, where creativity, passion,

compassion, and idealism have to struggle just to survive. This is the neoliberal grip from which it is difficult and for some even unthinkable to escape.

Authoritarian-Populist Reactions

For a small neoliberal city-state like Singapore, globalization has been viewed as offering not only the prospects of achieving prosperity through the expansion of trade and investment, but also the means of supplementing its limited human resources. Over the years, Singapore has been recording some of the lowest birth rates in the world, possibly exacerbated if not caused by lifestyle impotency from tiredness, stress, frustration, and anxiety over the ability to afford a good life in expensive Singapore (Emont, 2020). This has had deep implications for developing a workforce large enough to sustain Singapore's growth and development.

The people of this port-city, important even before colonial times, are today the product of generations of immigrants. In the 1970s, the government started to turn deliberately to migrants as a means of enlarging an inadequately proportioned workforce. This was meant to be only a temporary measure, until such time as Singapore's own people could expand and fill the gap or when technology and improved productivity could diminish the labour-intensive character of the construction, marine, and process sectors, among others. However, over the decades, Singapore's economy developed a dependency on low-waged and low-skilled workers from the region, whose widespread availability diminished the incentive to invest in productivity-enhancing technology and know-how. Pragmatic impatience and desire for instant results discouraged any deliberate measures that might be costly in the short term but necessary for long-term structural economic changes that could have weaned Singapore away from its migrant worker dependency. Instead, the number of imported migrant workers grew in an accelerated fashion after the mid-2000s when immigration policies were liberalized further.

At the other end of the migration spectrum is the so-called foreign talent category that includes foreigners who have qualifications and skills that Singapore believes it lacks and requires. Unlike low-waged migrant workers, considered to be "temporary" labourers who must eventually leave Singapore when they are no longer useful, internationally mobile foreign talents are highly paid and courted to live, work, and even take up citizenship in Singapore.

Today, out of a population of 5.8 million, there are almost a million migrant workers and less than 200,000 foreign talents. Their impact on the local population follows two main narratives. The more critical narrative points to how migrant workers, who are willing to work for very low wages, have the effect of suppressing the wages of the poorest Singaporeans, while the lifestyles of high-salaried foreign talents contribute to the increase in cost of living and the wage stagnation of middle-income Singaporeans. This—as well as the longer-term economic impact of technological change—explains the rise in income inequality, whose effects are inadequately mitigated by state welfare programmes that have been designed to prevent the poorest Singaporeans from becoming over-dependent on state assistance and support (Bhaskaran et al., 2012).

The second narrative draws upon the fundamentals of neoliberal globalization, asserting that even if many Singaporeans may feel that they are disadvantaged by liberal immigration policies, the presence of migrant workers keeps the cost of business and essential services affordable, especially for needier Singaporeans. Meanwhile, foreign talents help to create new jobs, transfer skills and know-how to local people, and shape the conditions for higher-order growth and development. This arrangement can improve the lives of all Singaporeans, as benefits trickle down to even the least advantaged among them. Moreover, many of the jobs that foreigners do, according to this neoliberal narrative, are jobs that Singaporeans either do not want to do or are unable to do well.

Neoliberal globalization and its prevailing explanatory narratives have not only been naturalized in an attempt to entrench them as the correct and only way of thinking, but they have also been obfuscated through the rhetoric of pragmatism. This is a deeply ideological manoeuvre, where the distinctive ideological position that is neoliberal globalization is first pervasively infused into the common sense of the people, and then disguised behind celebratory accounts of the Singapore approach to development, governance, and policymaking as non-ideological, even anti-ideological. Through a similar sleight of hand, it is critics of the government and the system who are instead cast as ideological and, in that sense, unrealistic, and even dangerous. Pragmatism has also erased ideological knowledge itself, so that most Singaporeans have little or no idea about the traditional ideological spectrum, what constitutes the beliefs, concerns, and aspirations of those on the left, right, and middle ground of that spectrum. Thus, in this vacuum of ideological knowledge, it has not been difficult to discredit and put away political opponents by characterizing them as Marxists, through a vulgar attempt to demonize using labels.

Singaporeans who may be experiencing dissatisfaction, social injustice, and unhappiness in their lives will likely have no alternative language for articulating it. Popular criticism therefore dwells within the logic of neoliberal globalization and rarely goes beyond the superficial and spectacular details of the neoliberal model, failing to reach the structurally deep levels that are the source of their problems and that require change. When public dissatisfaction with the debilitating effects of neoliberal globalization lacks theoretical and ideological sophistication, it accumulates, festers, and is exposed to manipulation by idealogues and demagogues.

Singapore is starting to see these developments and may be following in the footsteps of Donald Trump's America, where demagogues appeal to the unhappiness, hardship, and sense of righteousness of the aggrieved masses of left-behind Americans. By using instigative and inflammatory language, charismatic demagogues galvanize and channel these angry energies not towards the heart of neoliberal globalization, from which they in fact profit, but towards at least two visible targets. First is the establishment, made up of elites and their institutions that are described as out-of-touch, disdainful, corrupted, corrupting, and exploitative. Second are the minoritized communities who are portrayed as disloyal and immoral "others" within the nation, always a threat to national order and its way of life. This is essentially authoritarian populism, a perversion of democracy, which it often mimics grotesquely.

In a study of the United States, UK, and several European countries, US-based political scientists Pippa Norris and Ronald Inglehart (2019) concluded that the rise of contemporary populism in these places was mainly a reaction against social and cultural change and the increasing presence of immigrants in societies whose elites had embraced multiculturalism and cosmopolitanism. In pushing for greater tolerance of diversity and inclusion, these elites had in effect threatened the perspectives, values, and prospects of the once privileged majority. This has led to "cultural backlash", manipulated by charismatic leaders eager to gain political ascendancy by galvanizing a majoritarian sense of victimhood.

Similarly, UK-based political scientists Roger Eatwell and Matthew Goodwin (2018) explained what they called "national populism" as a "revolt against liberal democracy". They observed lower levels of trust in political institutions and the establishment, globalization's erosion of local community and identity, and neoliberal economics' exacerbation of inequality and deprivation, among others.

Harvard Professor Dani Rodrik (2017) argued that "right-wing" authoritarian populism was less a cultural backlash than it was a political reaction to the economic disruption and dislocation of globalization as it polarized the labour market and destroyed middle-class jobs. After decades of globalization, sizeable material gains have not been evenly distributed. Neoliberal elites—consisting of technocrats and the corporate elite—have benefitted considerably, while the rest have been severely disadvantaged, bearing the brunt of austerity measures implemented as neoliberal solutions to economic crises. Experiencing economic hardship, people become resentful of immigrants and other minorities, and receptive to populist parties and demagogues who tap into social undercurrents of xenophobia, racism, sexism, homophobia, ageism, and others to build support and distract from the very neoliberal policies from which they benefit.

Moral Panic

Authoritarian populist tendencies have started to emerge in Singapore as a reaction to the deleterious effects of an entrenched neoliberal globalization. One can expect to see more examples of moral panic, a classic sociological theory to explain a particular type of phenomenon observed in modern societies. Stanley Cohen's pioneering work on deviance and youth subcultures in the early 1970s still offers a useful working definition:

> Societies appear to be subject, every now and then, to periods of moral panic. A condition, episode, person, or group of persons emerges to become defined as a threat to societal values and interest; its nature is presented in stylized and stereotypical fashion by the mass media; the moral barricades are manned by editors, bishops, politicians, and other right thinking people; socially accredited experts pronounce their diagnosis and solutions; ways of coping are evolved or (more often) resorted to; the condition then disappears, submerges or deteriorates and becomes more visible. Sometimes the object of the panic is quite novel and at other times is something which has been in existence long enough, but suddenly appears in the limelight. Sometimes the panic passes over and is forgotten, except in folk lore and collective memory; at other times it has more serious and long-lasting repercussions and might produce such changes as those in

legal and social policy or even in the way society conceives itself. (Cohen, 1972)

One particularly useful formalization of moral panic emerged from the work of Erich Goode and Nachman Ben-Yahuda (1994) in the 1990s. They suggested that moral panic can be anatomized into a sequence of five elements or stages, each serving as criteria for identifying whether a moral panic has occurred.

The first of these elements is "concern". At this stage, one expects to see heightened public concern over a person or group, whose behaviour is viewed as a threat to the values and interests of mainstream society. The second element is "hostility", at which stage one expects to see a rise in the levels of hostility towards deviant groups, members of which are stylized as "folk devils", often through negative stereotypes in the mass media, in order to amplify deviance. The third element is "consensus" in mainstream society on the reality, extent, and cause of the threat, a consensus that is secured and reinforced by the combined efforts of politicians, religious leaders, news producers, experts, opinion leaders, and civil society activists who—through mass media platforms—form a moral barricade dividing "us" and "them". The fourth element is "disproportionality" between public reaction and reality. The fifth element is "volatility", the suddenness with which intense concern and hostility erupt and then recede, periodically. Though volatile, a moral panic can have lasting repercussions on culture and social-political institutions.

Volatile events reflecting mainstream society's heightened concern and hostility towards foreigners in Singapore—ranging from expressions of disgust to calls for surveillance—may be viewed as a symptom of latent and repressed feelings of anxiety, frustration, shame, denial, and even guilt over Singaporeans' complicity in exploitative practices towards migrant workers, the global-neoliberal basis upon which much of Singapore's success has been cheaply attained. In this sense, moral panic can be seen as symptomatic of an unhealthy body, straining to justify its exploitative pragmatism and thereby repress its conscience.

Perhaps more critically, moral panic over foreigners in Singapore may also be part of a larger policing mechanism for maintaining the hegemony of neoliberal globalization in times of crisis. Such a holistic analysis draws heavily on the ground-breaking critical theorization of Stuart Hall and his colleagues (1978) in the late 1970s. In their analysis of the significance of moral panic over young Afro-Caribbean "muggers" in Britain, they argued that consensus is quite complex, dynamic, and contested in modern capitalist society, even with the active complicity of the political elite, police, courts, legislature, and mass media. Broader ideological consensus, the basis of capitalist hegemony, is always a struggle to maintain, especially in times of crisis. Thus, manufacturing the spectacle of folk devils, the threat that they are thought to pose to mainstream society, and their consequent stigmatization and even "criminalization" helps to secure hegemony by creating the conditions within which it is easier to obtain broader consent and support. And through that fear-driven consent and active support, law-and-order politics and the culture of surveillance to "police the crisis" can be legitimized, elite interests protected, and the stability of the capitalist system restored with at most a tweaking of laws and regulations.

The very specific first-year effects of the COVID-19 pandemic in Singapore point to a crisis of neoliberal globalization. At such a time, one can expect to observe moral panic erupting out of authoritarian populist tendencies that have developed as a reaction to the excesses of neoliberal globalization over the last three decades or so. Indeed, when Singapore's infection rates increased, the immediate reaction was to define the problem as a migrant worker issue, isolate and subject them to heightened surveillance in their prison-like dormitories, and report their infection numbers separately from mainstream Singapore society or "community" where the problem in contrast seemed to be very much under control. In social media, many netizens pointed to migrant workers as the cause of infections in Singapore, drawing on stereotypes to paint images of cultural backwardness and lack of hygiene. Messages such as the following were widely circulated over private WhatsApp groups:

> 20,000 foreign workers are now quarantined in several large dormitories. If only 2 per cent are infected, they will infect onwards their maid girlfriends. We're talking 400 infected households. (Jaswal, 2020)

Even the mainstream media contributed to these kinds of narrative. A forum letter published in Chinese-language daily *Lianhe Zaobao*, for instance, suggested that foreign workers, their eating habits, and personal hygiene were likely to be the reasons for the infectious clusters. This drew the attention of a senior minister who described such views as racist and xenophobic (Aqil, 2020).

At the same time, though, there were others in social media who argued vigorously against the scapegoating of migrant worker folk devils. Local civil society organizations and activists also worked hard to advocate for the well-being of migrants who were trapped in their dormitories. Many, such as volunteers from Geylang Adventures, ItsRainingRaincoats, Singapore Migrant Friends, and Migrant X Me, banded together to form COVID Migrant Support Coalition. This informal group collected and distributed food and other useful items to the dormitories (Phua, 2020). Others, like the Humanitarian Organisation for Migration Economics (HOME) and Transient Workers Count Too (TWC2), kept a watchful eye on how the powerless were being treated by the powerful, reporting about liberties taken with regard to paying dormitory-bound workers the salaries they were entitled to, their basic freedoms and conditions of health (HOME and TWC2, 2021).

Eventually, the dormitory situation improved, and the pandemic seemed under control again. But the authoritarian populist reaction towards foreigners had the effect of drawing public attention away from not only questions about the government's competence, but also the larger crisis of capitalism that continues to confront the neoliberal global city. When Singapore eventually comes out of the pandemic crisis, its government will likely be in the strongest position to introduce new and enhanced modes of surveillance, intensifying its authoritarianism. But will this make Singapore more resilient?

Emerging from the Pandemic, Resilient?

The subsequent chapters in this book aim to address this question through different and yet thoroughly interconnected facets of the Singapore experience of governance and policymaking: The evolution of its neoliberalism, a history of its public health practices, its COVID-19 strategy, its immigration policies, and the migrant worker dormitory outbreaks.

In Chapter 2, Andrea Dugo describes how Singapore has come to embrace neoliberal globalization so tightly. He traces this to a pervasive and uncompromising ideology of survivalism, which was born in the early years of independence, after Singapore's expulsion from the Malaysian Federation in 1965. The notion of permanent vulnerability shaped the siege mentality of the newly formed city-state's ruling elite. This helped to justify its authoritarian politics, viewed as a protective, providential, and benign form of elite paternalism. However, instead of turning inwards, the leadership recognized how important it was for a small state with inadequate natural resources to be as connected to the world as possible. Therein lay its prospects for economic development and growth, which were in turn the bases of social stability, political legitimacy, and ultimately national survival in a dangerous world. In fully embracing a global-city identity and giving national primacy to economic growth and the role of markets for achieving it, Singapore had all the makings of a neoliberal global city from its early years of independence. After the mid-1980s, these neoliberal predilections eventually became imperatives. Neoliberal globalization has become the ultimate compass guiding the government's political action in virtually every field, from labour market and immigration policies, to public health policies. The partnership between neoliberal globalization and state authoritarianism has delivered impressive economic success, which has in turn inspired leaders of many other nations to emulate it. However, over the last two decades especially, the emergence of a number of problems, including those relating to income inequality and migrant workers, has revealed cracks in the system. The COVID-19 crisis has shed new light on these problems. Dugo argues that the pandemic is a moment of opportunity for Singapore to become a more inclusive society and thereby adapt to a future where neoliberal globalization itself will very likely be transformed, rather than destroyed.

In Chapter 3, Hongwu Lyu and Aymeric Vo Quang trace the development of Singapore's public health approaches by focusing on how its government dealt with tuberculosis, HIV/AIDS, and Severe Acute Respiratory Syndrome (SARS). These are historically significant cases of infectious disease outbreaks that have posed economic, social, reputational, and moral challenges to Singapore and its much-vaunted model. Lyu and Vo Quang trace the "exclusionary" aspect of neoliberalism in Singapore, arguing that, until only in recent years, Singapore's neoliberal public health system—focused on efficiency and optimal allocation—had neglected HIV/AIDS and thus the segments of society often associated with it. This neglect had been heightened by prevailing social stigmas and stereotypes. This may shed some light on the COVID-19 pandemic, which elicited rapid, responsive, robust, and inclusive government action where mainstream Singaporean community was concerned, but at the same time failed to recognize and deal with the marginalized and possibly stigmatized segments of society, such as migrant workers, whose badly infected dormitories became an international spectacle of crisis and social injustice. Lyu and Vo Quang draw on the example of tuberculosis to show how stigma attached to a disease, its sufferers, and their behaviours, and only partial public knowledge about these matters, had a direct effect on public intervention efficacy since colonial times. The COVID-19 crisis, in contrast, was managed somewhat differently. In an age of misinformation and disinformation, the government communicated frequently and transparently with the public, acknowledging uncertainty and gaps in their knowledge, but making clear what the scientific community were confident about. It did this in order to leave as little space for misinterpretation as possible. However, COVID-19 resembled tuberculosis and HIV/AIDS in terms of social stigmatization and even moral panic over the "unhealthy" elements in society. Teenage "spitters" who threatened to spread tuberculosis through their "defiant" behaviour, homosexuals who threatened to spread HIV/AIDS through their "immoral" behaviour, and migrant workers in dormitories who were the foreign bringers of disease were readily othered and viewed with disproportionate public concern and hostility. The SARS crisis in 2003, Lyu and Vo Quang argue, was a "wake-up call" for a less-than-prepared Singapore. They identify key lessons learnt by a subsequently more pro-active government, which were systematically institutionalized in readiness for the next infectious disease outbreak. The most unexpectedly challenging of these was to be COVID-19, 17 years later.

In Chapter 4, Johanna Dirlewanger-Lücke and Junhao Li describe how the Singapore government managed the COVID-19 crisis in its first year. The government's strategy, built upon its experience of handling the SARS crisis in 2003, showcased extensive capacities to test, trace, isolate, treat, and limit the importation of cases. Implementation was impressive at first, delivering results that were internationally admired. An emphasis on building social responsibility through transparent communication and the use of technology has also on the whole been successful. To keep the economy afloat and ready to thrive in post-pandemic times, the government allocated approximately $100 billion in a budget that was business- and employer-centric, consistent with neoliberal globalization. Where the government failed was in its handling of the disease outbreaks in migrant worker dormitories, which it seemed not to have anticipated even though there had been warnings from civil society activists. Opportunistically, the PAP called for early parliamentary elections, arguing that a PAP government with a strong mandate was what successful management of this "crisis of a generation" required. Since Singaporeans are often thought to be risk-averse, there was an expectation of a landslide victory for the PAP with voters taking a "flight to safety" and supporting the only government they had ever known in this dominant-party system. Instead, the PAP lost significant vote share and 10 seats including two multi-member "group representation constituencies" were lost to the opposition. If these results reflected what voters thought of the government's performance in managing the COVID-19 crisis, they may well point more specifically to public dissatisfaction with immigration policy and the dormitories fiasco.

In Chapter 5, Davide Brugola and Michael Flood trace the roots of immigration policy in cosmopolitan Singapore, today marked by separate flows of foreign talent and migrant workers. They discuss how the PAP government's pragmatic, which has come to really mean dogmatically neoliberal, approach to immigration policy has been shaped by the Great Recession of 2007–2009, relatively disappointing results in the 2011 general elections, and popular reactions to a 2013 population white paper that pointed to a more crowded future with greater numbers of foreigners in the global city. Brugola and Flood argue that, in response to popular pressure against excessive inflow of foreigners, the government tends to express empathy in public communication and make marginal revisions to the policy, while adamantly pursuing a neoliberal agenda that keeps Singapore profitably reliant on foreign labour. The "Little India riot", which exploded in a crowded district where South Asian migrant workers congregated on their days off, pointed to the untenability of this policy approach. And yet, not much has changed subsequently, leading to the vivid exposure of the system's vulnerability when it was confronted with an unexpected global public health crisis in 2020.

In Chapter 6, Carolin Bernhard and Mara Ellemunt discuss the many dimensions of precarity that Singapore's migrant workers experience, particularly as it pertains to the question of space. In neoliberal Singapore, capitalism thrives on the exploitation of low-waged migrant workers who are attracted to Singapore to earn a living building and cleaning the city and serving its residents. Their presence in this already crowded city provokes a dualistic public response that originates from a grudging acceptance of their indispensability: on the one hand, a refusal to allow them to fully integrate with Singapore society and be treated as equal human beings; and, on the other hand, a compassionate desire to help them when they are in need. The former tendency has had the effect of making migrant workers as invisible as possible, hence the profitable solution to house large numbers of them in dormitories located in the peripheral spaces of the island. Capitalism, profit maximization, and space optimization have created conditions and practices of exploitation that are, in normal times, cloaked in invisibility. The 2020 outbreak of COVID-19 in these dormitory spaces should hardly be surprising, unless they had been so well hidden in the blind spots of public conscience and policy consciousness. The outbreaks also produced dualistic public reactions: moral panic and the stigmatization of infectious foreigners as dirty and dangerous folk devils, which demands further spatial segregation; and civic activism that steps up to the service of helping the vulnerable in their time of need. Bernhard and Ellemunt suggest that the solutions going forward will likely be technical rather than normative in nature, well within the segregating and exploitative logic of neoliberal globalization, with ever-more-ingenious ways to extract value from migrant worker labour, whilst making them and the heterotopia in which they exist as invisible and distant as possible.

The Singapore government—clean, elite, and pragmatic—has been a successful government, leading a remarkable transformation of this small post-colonial country of limited size and resources into a prosperous, safe, and liveable city for a peaceful, meritocratic, and multi-ethnic society. Since the 1980s, however, this same government has become increasingly attached to a way of thinking that is tightly associated with the logic and values of the market. The pragmatism of an earlier time has hardened into a dogmatic, almost fundamentalist, adherence to efficiency and economic growth as proper ends in themselves. Bold, far-sighted policies aimed at transforming Singapore to meet the known and unknown challenges of an increasingly volatile, uncertain, complex, and ambiguous world are no longer to be found in the establishment, where the political heroes of the independence generation have given way to technocrats very mindful of, and limited by, their careers and egos. In such a brittle condition, how resilient can Singapore be?

References

Aqil Hafiz Mahmud (2020) "COVID-19: Forum letter on foreign worker dormitory cases reveals 'underlying racism', says Shanmugam", *Channel News Asia*, 18 April.

Bhaskaran, Manu et al. (2012) "Inequality and the need for a new social compact", Singapore Perspectives 2012 conference. Institute of Policy Studies.

Cai, Weiyi and K.K. Rebecca Lai (2020) "Packed with migrant workers, dormitories fuel Coronavirus in Singapore", *The New York Times*, 28 April.

Chew, Hui Min (2021) "Will air travel bubbles take off or burst?", *Channel News Asia*, 21 March.

Cohen, Stanley (1972) *Folk Devils and Moral Panics: The Creation of the Mods and Rockers*, MacGibbon and Kee.

Eatwell, Roger and Matthew Goodwin (2018) *National Populism: The Revolt Against Liberal Democracy*, Pelican.

Economist Intelligence Unit (2020) "Worldwide Cost of Living 2020: Which global cities have the highest cost of living?"

Emont, Jon (2020) "Singapore isn't kidding when it comes to fostering fertility", *The Wall Street Journal*, 22 February.

Giroux, Henry A. (2004) *The Terror of Neoliberalism: Authoritarianism and the Eclipse of Democracy*, Routledge.

Glasgow, Will (2020) "Coronavirus: Hibernation v elimination, it all comes down to culture", *The Australian*, 4 April.

Goode, Erich and Nachman Ben-Yahuda (1994) *Moral Panics: The Social Construction of Deviance*, Wiley-Blackwell.

Hall, Stuart, Chas Critcher, Tony Jefferson, John Clarke, and Bryan Roberts (1978) *Policing the Crisis: Mugging, The State, and Law and Order*, Macmillan.

Harvey, David (2005) *A Brief History of Neoliberalism*, Oxford University Press.

Heng, Cheryl and Bonnie Au (2021) "One year into COVID-19 pandemic, world marks anniversary of WHO's declaration on coronavirus", Video, *South China Morning Post*, 11 March. https://www.scmp.com/video/cor onavirus/3125018/one-year-covid-19-pandemic-world-marks-anniversary-whos-declaration.

HOME and TWC2 (2021) "Migrant workers in Singapore: An update", *FOCUS Asia-Pacific*, Asia-Pacific Human Rights Information Center, Vol. 104, June.

Jaswal, Balli Kaur (2020) "Rise in coronavirus cases brings to light Singaporeans' racist attitudes towards foreign workers", *South China Morning Post*, 23 April.

Kisi (2020) "Cities with the best work-life balance 2020". https://www.getkisi.com/work-life-balance-2020.

Leung, Hillary (2020) "Singapore was a Coronavirus success story—Until an outbreak showed how vulnerable workers can fall through the cracks", *Time*, 29 April.

Norris, Pippa and Ronald Inglehart (2019) *Cultural Backlash: Trump, Brexit, and Authoritarian Populism*, Cambridge University Press.

Phua, Rachel (2020) "NGOs launch initiatives to help migrant workers amid COVID-19 outbreak", *Channel News Asia*, 10 April.

Rajaratnam, S. (1972) "Singapore: Global city", speech at Singapore Press Club dinner, 6 February.

Ratcliffe, Rebecca (2020) "Singapore's cramped migrant worker dorms hide Covid-19 surge risk", *The Guardian*, 17 April.

Rodrik, Dani (2017) *Straight Talk on Trade: Ideas for a Sane World Economy*, Princeton University Press.

Roozenbeek, Jon et al. (2020) "Susceptibility to misinformation about COVID-19 around the world", *Royal Society Open Science*, 7(10). https://royalsoci etypublishing.org/doi/full/10.1098/rsos.201199.

Sandel, Michael (2012) *What Money Can't Buy: The Moral Limits of Markets*, Farrar, Straus, and Giroux.

Sassen, Saskia (1991) *The Global City: New York, London, Tokyo*, Princeton University Press.

Scholte, Jan Aart (2005) "The sources of neoliberal globalization", Overarching Concerns Programme Paper Number 8, October, United Nations Research Institute for Social Development.

Schwab, Klaus (2015) "The fourth industrial revolution: What it means and how to respond", *Foreign Affairs*, 12 December.

Smith, Catherine J. et al. (2015) *A Handbook on Inequality, Poverty and Unmet Social Needs in Singapore*. Social Insight Research Series. Lien Centre for Social Innovation.

Tan, Kenneth Paul (2017) *Governing Global-City Singapore: Legacies and Futures after Lee Kuan Yew*, Routledge.

Tan, Kenneth Paul (2018) *Singapore: Identity, Brand, Power*, Cambridge University Press.

Tan, Shu Yan (2018) "Sleep deprivation still a problem in work-oriented, fast-paced Singapore", *The Straits Times*, 3 April.

Toh, Ting Wei (2020) "Unilateral reopening of borders a small, cautious step to revive Changi: Ong", *The Straits Times*, 22 August.

UN News (2021) "COVID-19: Virus variants, vaccine inequity, contribute to rising caseload", 19 March.

"WHO praises Singapore's response to coronavirus outbreak" (2020) *The Straits Times*, 19 February.

World Health Organization (2017) "Depression and other common mental disorders: Global health estimates". https://apps.who.int/iris/bitstream/han dle/10665/254610/WHO-MSD-MER-2017.2-eng.pdf.

Young, Jin Yu (2021) "In lockdown for 18 months, Singapore's migrant workers yearn for freedom". *The New York Times*, 29 September.

CHAPTER 2

Neoliberal Singapore: Nation-State and Global City

Andrea Dugo

Abstract Singapore has come to embrace neoliberal globalization very tightly due to a pervasive and uncompromising ideology of survivalism, which was born in the early years of independence, after Singapore's expulsion from the Malaysian Federation in 1965. The notion of permanent vulnerability shaped the siege mentality of the newly formed city-state's ruling elite. This helped to justify its authoritarian politics, viewed as a protective, providential, and benign form of elite paternalism. However, instead of turning inwards, the leadership recognized how important it was for a small state with inadequate natural resources to be as connected to the world as possible. Therein lay its prospects for economic development and growth, which were in turn the bases of social stability, political legitimacy, and ultimately national survival in a dangerous world. In fully embracing a global-city identity and giving national primacy to economic growth and the role of markets for

A. Dugo (✉)
Double Master Degree in Public Policy and European Affairs, National University of Singapore and Sciences Po (2021), Corsico, Italy
e-mail: e04040694@u.nus.edu; andrea.dugo@sciencespo.fr

© The Author(s), under exclusive license to Springer Nature Singapore Pte Ltd. 2022
K. P. Tan (ed.), *Singapore's First Year of COVID-19*,
https://doi.org/10.1007/978-981-19-0368-7_2

23

achieving it, Singapore had all the makings of a neoliberal global city from its early years of independence. After the mid-1980s, these neoliberal predilections eventually became imperatives. Neoliberal globalization has become the ultimate compass guiding the government's political action in virtually every field, from labour market and immigration policies, to public health policies. The partnership between neoliberal globalization and state authoritarianism has delivered impressive economic success, which has in turn inspired leaders of many other nations to emulate it. However, over the last two decades especially, the emergence of several problems, including those relating to income inequality and migrant workers, has revealed cracks in the system. The COVID-19 crisis has shed new light on these problems. The pandemic is a moment of opportunity for Singapore to become a more inclusive society and thereby adapt to a future where neoliberal globalization itself will very likely be transformed, rather than destroyed.

Keywords Survival · Nation-state · Global city · Economic growth · Authoritarianism · Pandemic crisis · Inclusive society

SURVIVAL AND THE SIEGE MENTALITY

Whenever its governing elite is asked to explain Singapore, an adjective that nearly always emerges is "vulnerable". From the time Singapore gained independence in 1965, the ruling class has continuously stressed the intrinsic vulnerability of the country as a small city-state and has consequently built around it a deeply entrenched siege mentality and a strong sense of national identity (Magcamit, 2015; Heng, 2013; Chang, 2019).

Former head of the Singapore Civil Service, Peter Ho, rightly points out that the vulnerability mantra is not an exclusive prerogative of Singapore.

> [All] sovereign city states are anomalies, surviving despite their very small size, without natural resource, and surrounded by much larger neighbours. Their existence is a constant struggle with challenges that larger nations

with hinterlands and resources do not worry about. They are a paradox, the exceptions that prove the rule that size matters. (Ho, 2018: 77)

The ruling elite has cultivated and inculcated in citizens a deeply embedded siege mentality, the basis of something like a national philosophy. It is no wonder that, when Singapore's former ambassador to the United States, Chan Heng Chee, was asked what she thought was Singapore's first Prime Minister Lee Kuan Yew's most significant legacy to the country, she promptly replied that it was to have "thought through and implemented a strategy of small state survival" (Guo and Woo, 2013). There are indeed strong grounds to understand why Singapore has developed such a tight fortress mentality. When the city-state gained independence in 1965 after its ejection from the Malaysian Federation, very few thought that Singapore could survive. Less than a decade earlier, in fact, Lee (1957) himself had declared that "island-nations [were] political jokes". When it achieved independence in the mid-1960s, Singapore suffered from an array of pre-existing conditions that characterize many small developing island-states, among which were rapid population growth, job shortages, deep ethnic cleavages, and scarcity of natural endowments (Chew, 2000). To these, the absence of a natural hinterland, the lack of a large domestic market, and "military pressure from potentially hostile neighbors" (Heng, 2013: 437) must also be added. In other words, all odds seemed stacked against Singapore.

The most viable way for a small state to navigate the Hobbesian anarchy of turbulent international waters and come out of them unscathed was to espouse, as the ruling elite continues to do, an ideology of "survivalism",

which specifically stressed the lack of national identity, the absence of a viable national economy and the vulnerability of the society to international and internal threats. They sought legitimacy by inculcating a siege mentality in which it was precisely the lack of state power and of national cohesion which made political acquiescence by civil society so imperative. (Brown, 1998: 39)

Survivalism is, in fact, an attitude of perpetual emergency that places maximum focus on national protection from all internal and external threats to a country's survival. In Singapore, this "garrison mentality" has been a potent catalyst for forging a common sense of nationhood across a multiracial society ever since independence (Tan, 2001: 97). Framing nationhood in terms of collectively facing ever-present existential risks and threats has proved a useful narrative for the government to rally mass support, forge national cohesion, and build a common identity.

THE GLOBAL CITY

The flipside of what could seem like parochial survivalist rhetoric was in fact an outward focus on connecting to the world. For a small country like Singapore, survivalism could not simply equate with barricading inside city-state borders. Small state survival can only be ensured in an international environment that is primed to be as favourable as possible.

In the words of Lee Kuan Yew (2009),

A small country must seek a maximum number of friends, while maintaining the freedom to be itself as a sovereign and independent nation. ... We must make ourselves relevant so that other countries have an interest in our continued survival and prosperity as a sovereign and independent nation. Singapore cannot take its relevance for granted. Small countries perform no vital or irreplaceable functions in the international system. Singapore has to continually reconstruct itself and keep its relevance to the world and to create political and economic space. This is the economic imperative for Singapore.

To survive and thrive as a small state, Singapore's future depended profoundly on the international order. Since the late 1960s, "the major state strategy for strengthening the nation-state was that of globalisation" (Brown, 1998: 39). By opening up to the world, Singapore's political elite endeavoured to make the island-nation an indispensable piece of the emerging international economic puzzle. If Singapore needed the world, the world needed to need Singapore. This is when the global city strategy made its stage appearance.

First to characterize Singapore's quest to become a global city as a matter of life and death for the city-state was its Foreign Affairs Minister, S. Rajaratnam. As early as 1972, a mere seven years since independence, he laid out his vision for a global Singapore in a famous speech to the Singapore Press Club.

A small city state, without a natural hinterland, without a large domestic market and no raw materials to speak of, has a near-zero chance of survival politically, economically or militarily. … But once you see Singapore as a Global City the problem of hinterland becomes unimportant because *for a Global City the world is its hinterland*. … There are admittedly grave political and economic dangers implicit in the entry of powerful foreign concerns into weak and underdeveloped countries. … But Singapore must be prepared to undertake these risks simply because the alternative to not moving into the global economic system is, for a small Singapore, *certain death*. … An independent Singapore survives and will survive because it has established a relationship of interdependence in the rapidly expanding global economic system. Singapore's economic future will, as the years go by, become more and more rooted in this global system. *It will grow and prosper as this system grows and prospers. It will collapse if this system collapses.* (Rajaratnam, 1972: 2, 8, 11–12, emphasis added)

In the ruling People's Action Party's (PAP) narrative, if Singapore could not achieve global status, it would simply cease to exist. By this logic, Singapore opened itself to international business. The attraction of foreign capital, along with the transformation of Singapore into a world-class aviation hub and maritime centre, became priorities at the top of the PAP agenda (Heng, 2013). Openness to international markets was seen as not only a matter of survival; it was also the most effective way to bring about widespread economic prosperity. According to this line of thought, as the whole-hearted adoption of market principles would rapidly elevate Singapore from a regional trading post to a global financial capital, the benefits of this metamorphosis would percolate down to the entire population and improve living standards for all (Brown, 1998).

Economic performance thus became the ultimate baseline of Singaporean policymaking. By promising to deliver on robust economic performance, the PAP regime would fulfil the twofold goal of ensuring national cohesion internally and securing Singapore as a safe place internationally (Dent, 2001). The PAP government came to view the pursuit of economic prosperity as its ultimate source of legitimacy and as the only viable solution to the question of survival.

AUTHORITARIAN NEOLIBERALISM

In the PAP's narrative, the achievement of successful capitalistic development was the only way to keep the spectre of Singapore's vulnerability at bay. "Economicism" thus became synonymous with survivalism. For Singapore to survive, all societal efforts needed to be directed towards fostering economic growth (Wang, 2012). Economic performance became Singapore's civic religion.

Singapore's obsession with the primacy of capitalist economics is by no means surprising nor unique. The rise of neoliberalism is often traced back to the late 1970s, when Margaret Thatcher in the United Kingdom and Ronald Reagan in the United States began pursuing path-breaking policies of extreme economic liberalization. The tendency to subordinate all aspects of policymaking to the economic competitiveness fetish has become virtually universal. David Harvey (2005: 2–3) asserted that:

> There has everywhere been an emphatic turn towards neoliberalism in political-economic practices and thinking since the 1970s. Deregulation, privatization, and withdrawal of the state from many areas of social provision have been all too common. ... Neoliberalism has, in short, become hegemonic as a mode of discourse ... [when seeking] to bring all human action into the domain of the market.

What sets Singapore apart, though, is how early on it embraced "neoliberal" principles, at the very least an obsession with economics and markets. Singapore's "economy first" doctrine for the survival of a small state has prompted scholars to ask whether it has in fact been neoliberal ever since 1965. US-based scholars Narumi Naruse and Weihsin Gui (2016: 476) for instance suggest:

> If pro-business state intervention is an early sign of economic neoliberalization, then this mode of governance had its beginnings in Singapore .... Our intention is not to claim Singapore as an originating centre of neoliberalism but to show ... [that] Singapore's early years of independence anticipate neoliberal formations.

Such a claim does not necessarily erase Singapore's "social democratic" phase, at least in its earlier years as an independent nation. Forged as a social democratic party in the mid-1950s, the PAP pursued social justice-oriented policies from the very outset of its rule, among which included a large-scale national public housing programme and public controls on capital (Chua, 2019). However, the PAP's original social democratic adherence proved short-lived. Traditionally social democratic impulses, such as trade unionism and labour mobilization, were systematically stifled in the cradle not only because of mounting fear over a spread of Communism in the city-state, but also in the ultimate interest of Singapore's economic competitiveness (Luther, 1979). Although the independent Singapore of today bears features that are traceable to its social democratic starting points, such as heavy state presence in and control of the economy, Singapore has in effect separated from social democracy, embracing neoliberalism instead as its new mistress to achieve the ecstasy of economic growth.

Singapore's relationship with neoliberalism has been a long and enduring one. The peculiarity behind this successful relationship resides in the unique ability of the PAP regime to strike the right balance between economic freedom and political and civil repression. This is no sole prerogative of Singapore. Other countries, from Chile to Russia, have attempted to combine authoritarian rule with neoliberalism (Letelier, 1976; Rutland, 2013). However, the Singaporean variety of authoritarian neoliberalism is one of the few genuine success stories and by far the longest lasting one. The secret to this accomplishment, many scholars think, is to be found in the PAP's cleverness in putting the survivalist narrative at the service of authoritarian neoliberalism. Bloom (2016: 84), for instance, argues that, "the persistent authoritarian refrain of survival and preservation deployed by the PAP … represents the resiliency of neoliberal discourses of authoritarian modernization". By bringing about and safeguarding economic growth and, most importantly, by framing it as a matter of life and death for the city-state, the PAP's dominant-party rule is made indispensable or, at the very least, palatable.

PRAGMATISM, ELITISM, AND PATERNALISM

A widespread siege mentality offers Singapore's ruling elite the chance to frame every threat as existential and every proposed solution as unquestionable. According to Wang (2012: 372), "Singaporeans have been constantly reminded of the vulnerability of their nation, … which justifies the state's developmental strategies and its embrace of globalization". The basic assumption is that the PAP government knows what is best for the Singaporean people and always makes the best decisions and crafts the best policies in every circumstance.

Such a paternalistic conception of state management is once again a legacy of Singapore's early years of sovereign statehood. When independence was forced upon Singapore in 1965, the PAP found itself in charge of a small and ethnically polarized city-state, prone to riots and social instability (Garfinkle, 2020). Fearful that social unrest could undermine the survival of the newborn island-nation, the PAP government prioritized public orderliness and set out to steer the country in the most paternalistic way. By stepping in and regulating virtually all fields of civic life, the government continually attempts to craft a cohesive, state-imposed national identity (Teo, 2014). Policy decisions are centralized, roughly discarding inconvenient alternative perspectives, while paying full attention to results rather than process. The government has described this outcome-focused style of policymaking as "pragmatic". This ubiquitous word has been used to describe Singapore's supposedly ideology-free approach to every policy field, from foreign policy to LGBT issues.

One manifestation of Singapore-style pragmatism is the solving of existing problems by copying best practices from around the world and applying them without any ideological preconception. As Kishore Mahbubani (2010: 37), prominent Singaporean diplomat and former dean of the Lee Kuan Yew School of Public Policy, put it,

> policymakers do not adopt approaches that are driven by any ideology or intellectual framework. Instead their goal is to focus on results. And if an approach works to enhance security, it is adopted, even if it may appear to be intellectually incoherent or contradictory. At the end of the day, Deng Xiaoping's wise maxim describes contemporary East Asian approaches to security: "It does not matter whether a cat is black or white; if it catches mice, it is a good cat".

However, no matter how neutral and purely results-driven Singapore-style pragmatism purports to be, it has taken on a highly elitist and, quite ironically, ideological connotation. In the framework of Singaporean politics, pragmatism equates with the unrestrained pursuit of economic growth as "the singular criterion for initiating and assessing all government activities, in terms of how an act will aid or retard this growth" (Chua, 1995: 68). With the justification that economic growth is to be achieved at all costs, the PAP reserves itself the right to decide what policies are in the best interest of the country and to silence dissent around these policies by attaching the "pragmatic" label to them. Pragmatic policymaking is thus reduced to a starkly technocratic and elitist exercise of power. According to this logic, by keeping the goal of economic competitiveness above all others, pragmatism helps perpetuate the PAP's pro-business agenda, on the one hand, caressing the interests of international capital and, on the other, putting a curb on adverse social forces, thus furthering the party's position in power (Tan, 2017).

By providing the PAP regime with a handy, all-purpose narrative to justify its rule, Singapore's pragmatism thus serves to reinforce neoliberalism and authoritarianism concurrently (Wee, 2012). And it is precisely at the confluence of these three "isms"—pragmatism, neoliberalism, and authoritarianism—that the Singaporean model of governance thrives. This unique combination thus makes Singapore a *sui generis* neoliberal state. As David Harvey (2005: 86) put it,

> The case of Singapore is particularly instructive. It has combined neoliberalism in the marketplace with draconian coercive and authoritarian state power, while invoking moral solidarities based on the nationalist ideals of a beleaguered island state …, Confucian values, and, most recently, a distinctive form of the cosmopolitan ethic suited to its current position in the world of international trade.

The Persistent Centrality of the State

What sets Singapore's apart from other forms of neoliberalism, and thus makes it a seductive model for non-Western countries to follow, is the persistent centrality of government. Neoliberalism in the West has been almost always associated with the retreat of the state from the economic sphere. Whether it be measured by the level of subsidies, the number of state-owned enterprises, or the rate of capital taxation, all major policy indicators point to the incontrovertible fact that, since the 1980s, state intervention in the economy has been rolled back in virtually all advanced Western democracies (Zohlnhöfer et al., 2018).

This widespread development can be traced to the Thatcherite conviction that to promote societal efficiency, governments should step aside and let market forces prevail. Singapore was not immune to this megatrend. The PAP regime responded to the global influence of Thatcherism in the 1990s by altering its long-held paternalistic approach to state management. Top civil servant Peter Ho (2018: 84) observed how his government began investigating ways to step back and make way for the animal spirits of the private sector to rise, proceeding to privatize a number of state-owned companies, starting with Singapore Telecoms in 1993 and then liberalizing the telecommunications industry. In terms of fiscal policy, the corporate tax rate was lowered from 40% before 1987 to the currently capped 18% (Peng and Phang, 2018: 36).

However, unlike in many Western countries, the rolling back of the state was somewhat cosmetic in Singapore. One would have expected the numerous state-owned enterprises, known as government-linked companies (GLCs) in Singapore, to be the primary and most natural target of a comprehensive post-1990s neoliberal process of privatization and state rescaling. On the surface, the state did reduce its direct involvement in former GLCs. Some of them, such as Singapore Telecommunications, Singapore Post, and Singapore's Post Office Savings Bank, have formally been privatized (Heracleous, 2001; Low, 2002a; Tay, 2019). However, despite their independent status, most of these companies still maintain solid relations with the government. As such, the Singaporean state is far from being a disinterested former owner, but instead acts as the de facto supervisor and coordinator of the operations of these officially private companies (Liow, 2012: 249). Former GLCs are the continuation of state power by other means.

The government's firm, albeit more indirect, control over former state-owned enterprises remains as strong as ever and is much more reminiscent of plain old state dirigisme rather than neoliberal-inspired private enterprise. In stark contrast with the Western model of neoliberalism, the Singaporean government has managed to substantially preserve its central role in the economy while, at the same time, letting the entrepreneurial energies of local and international capitalism run rampant. As Nathan Peng and Sock Yong Phang (2018: 33) explain,

> The chief paradox of Singapore's growth story is the strong hand of government in directing free markets without compromising the market, and without the perceived ills that often come with government intervention, suggesting that a strong government and a well-functioning market are not a dichotomy.

The Singaporean model of a strong—even authoritarian—state, with a firm hand on the economic reins, serves as an alluring alternative for countries wishing to embrace non-Western varieties of neoliberalism. It will come as no surprise to learn that one of the greatest admirers of Singapore's approach to economic development was China's Deng Xiaoping (Ho, 2018: 78). On his famous "southern tour" in 1992, Deng spoke words of appreciation for Singapore's ability to combine good governance, the maintenance of social order, and a lively economic environment. The Chinese fascination with Singapore's development experience has even prompted some scholars to assert that the much talked about "Beijing Consensus" (Cooper Ramo, 2004), that is China's allegedly replicable model of authoritarian state-capitalism as opposed to the Western archetype of free-market democracy based on the Washington Consensus, is nothing other than a revisited Singapore model (Ortmann, 2012).

A Corporate Style of State Management

The main reason why the strong state in Singapore has been able to emerge virtually unscathed from the wave of "roll-back neoliberalism" (Birch and Mykhnenko, 2009) of the 1980s and 1990s is that the state was neoliberal to begin with. The government did not need to make space for private companies to step in and take care of public services on its behalf because the state in Singapore is itself run much like a company. As early as 1974, Louis Kraar (1974), Asia correspondent for *Fortune*, described Singapore this way:

> Singapore has achieved this dazzling growth by stretching its meager means and using some extraordinary techniques of statecraft. The country is run very much like a corporation. Striving above all for efficiency, the government coldly weighs every move, from school curriculums to foreign relations, against cost-effectiveness. The key criterion, as one top-rank official puts it, is always: "What good can we get out of it?"

Kraar's account of Singapore as a company-like country is no anomaly. At different times in recent history, a number of commentators have stressed the peculiarly entrepreneurial style of state management that characterizes its government. American author William Gibson (1993), notorious for dubbing the island-country a "Disneyland with the death penalty", wrote that the Singapore state "has the look and feel of a very large corporation. If IBM had ever bothered to actually possess a physical country, that country might have had a lot in common with Singapore". Similarly, American futurist Peter Schwartz (2010) described Singapore as "the Apple of nations". The PAP regime itself takes pride in likening Singapore to a company. In his 2010 National Day Rally speech, Prime Minister Lee Hsien Loong (2010) famously declared that "Microsoft is

... the kind of business which we want to be as Singapore". High-profile public officials often like to refer to the city-state as "Singapore Inc" (Lee, 2007).

The Singapore ministerial cabinet is thus like the country's board of directors. Its policies are like marketable products. Its citizens are like consumers. National identity is tied to economic profitability. By drawing national pride from economic growth, the PAP regime inevitably reinforces Singapore's metaphor of the nation-corporation "with a product to sell and a brand to protect" (Singh, 2019: 162). As a result, the government indissolubly binds the concept of Singaporeanness with the country's economic status. Far from being just a sterile macroeconomic box to tick, Singapore's economic competitiveness comes to be a vivid testament to the city-state's world-class reputation and the ultimate cornerstone of national identity.

Singapore's government handles policy issues in the most managerial fashion. It mathematically evaluates the tangible benefits and costs of every choice. It seeks to attract to its ranks the most talented Singaporeans, rewarding them according to their performance. It frames the official narrative through the language of business. All aspects of policymaking are rigorously examined with a neoliberal lens and the bottom line remains the primary, sometimes only, guiding principle behind government action. This highly corporate approach to public policymaking culminated in the public sector managerial reforms of the 1990s—collectively termed Public Service for the 21st Century (PS21)—which were led by then Head of Civil Service Lim Siong Guan. Broadly in line with the then-globally dominant doctrine of New Public Management, which set out to improve public service performance by introducing mechanisms of market discipline (Hill and Varone, 2017: 330), the PS21 reforms were envisaged to prioritize efficiency over equity in public service provision and to increase the accountability of civil servants (*The Straits Times*, 1995). In essence, PS21 attempted to make the public sector even more like the private sector.

Labour Market Policy. This corporate mentality in the public sector can be found in labour market policymaking. As early as the 1960s, in an effort to attract large-scale foreign investment, the PAP government sought to rid Singapore of its reputation as a labour dispute and strike-prone country. Then-President Yusof bin Ishak said, "the excesses of irresponsible trade unions ... are luxuries which we can no longer afford"

(LePoer, 1989: 59). To this end, the PAP passed the Industrial Relations Act, which irremediably crippled the bargaining power of organized labour and rendered strikes unlawful if not authorized by the government (Naruse and Gui, 2016). In 1968, the bill was amended once again to favour multinational corporations, by making it "an offence for a trade union to raise for collective bargaining matters pertaining to the promotion, transfer, hiring, firing or job allocation of an employee" (Leggett, 2005: 107), thus further constraining the workers' negotiating power. The labour laws introduced in the late 1960s massively enhanced job creation in the city-state by producing an efficient, cheap, and pliant workforce, making Singapore an attractive destination for transnational companies in pursuit of low-cost country sourcing (Han and Seng, 2014).

Ever since then, labour market legislation has prioritized the profits of the Singaporean nation-corporation over citizens' working conditions. As Singaporean sociologist Chua Beng Huat (1995: 18) put it, "the sectional interest of labour was … subjugated to the larger interest of national survival". Even in more recent years, labour market policy has kept on being filtered through a neoliberal prism of decision-making. For instance, the PAP regime has fiercely resisted all calls for the introduction of a minimum wage on the basis that an increase in the cost of labour would most likely drive international businesses away and thus hurt the country's competitiveness. In 2004, in response to widespread calls for a minimum wage, the Ministry of Manpower declared, "whether wages should increase or decrease is best determined by market demand and supply for labour, skills, capabilities and competency to perform the task" (Hooi, 2004). In 2009, Lee Kuan Yew himself weighed in on the issue and claimed that "every country that has set a minimum wage over what the market will bear has found that the move cuts jobs" (Au Yong, 2009).

In a similar spirit, the introduction of a cash pay-out scheme for low-wage and elderly workers in 2007, the so-called Workfare Income Supplement (WIS) scheme, was conceived not as a disinterested form of income support for the worst-off in society, but in strict accordance with a neoliberal logic of self-reliance, as conditional on their participation in the labour force. What the WIS scheme effectively illustrates is the government-sponsored idea that citizens, regardless of age, always need to take charge of their own welfare. They must not feel entitled to government aid. And they must be in active employment to qualify for it (Liow, 2012).

Immigration Policy. Immigration policy is indissolubly connected with labour market issues. Over the decades, the PAP regime has crafted a constellation of policies to regulate a growing number of immigrants in search of employment in Singapore. To manage this increasing inflow, the government put in place a Work Pass system, created in the early 1980s and reviewed in the late 1990s, that distinguishes among migrant workers based on their class, education level, and ethnicity (Liow, 2012).

Singapore's immigrants are broadly classified as either foreign talents or foreign workers. The first are desired as highly educated and highly skilled workers who can contribute considerably to the economic development of the city-state in a number of fields, ranging from biomedicine to finance to academia. Since the 1990s, fearful of competition from other global cities and grasping the ever-increasing importance of high-quality human capital for the emerging knowledge-based economy, the government has been endeavouring to render the city-state a talent capital (Low, 2002b). The rhetoric of drawing foreign talents to Singapore has thus become central in the official PAP discourse. Former Prime Minister Goh Chok Tong (2002) declared that "attracting international talent to Singapore ... is crucial for our growth and development". Lee Kuan Yew (2003) once made it clear that "if we do not attract, welcome and make foreign talent feel comfortable in Singapore, we will not be a global city and if we are not a global city, it doesn't count for much".

At the other end of the spectrum are low-skilled and semi-qualified foreign workers. Due to local shortages of low-skilled workers, the PAP regime has viewed the inflow of foreign workers as indispensable. Foreign workers are a mere economic tool for Singapore's survival, only permitted entry into the city-state to erect the necessary infrastructure, clean the city, and serve the needs of native Singaporeans and foreign talents. In essence, their function is simply to ensure the basic working of the Singaporean economy (Liow, 2012).

The two-tiered nature of the Singaporean immigration system is one of the most emblematic examples of the PAP's corporate take on policymaking. Liow (2012: 254) argues that the Work Pass system, which discriminates so blatantly between foreign talents and foreign workers and hence assigns them a starkly differential immigration treatment, "is an outcome of the desire of the Singapore neoliberal-developmental state to create and sustain economic growth in the most economically efficient and 'pragmatic' manner possible". Foreign talents, with the potential to contribute greatly to the country's long-term economic growth, are given white-glove treatment and are thus offered extremely beneficial terms to lure them to the city-state and persuade them to make it their home. At the other end of the spectrum, foreign workers, whose potential contribution to economic prosperity is much more limited in scope, are made use of for however long is needed and eventually sent back to their home countries, having virtually zero chances of staying in Singapore as permanent residents or, even less, of acquiring citizenship.

MARKET MORALITY

To the ruling elite, even decisions taken in the privacy of one's personal life should ultimately serve the purpose of boosting economic growth. In this respect, Lee Kuan Yew (1986, video at 3:46, 29:51, and 31:20) once famously said:

> I am accused often of interfering in the private lives of citizens. Yes, if I did not, had I not done that, we wouldn't be here today. ... And I say without the slightest remorse, that we wouldn't be here, we would not have made economic progress, if we had not intervened on very personal matters – who your neighbour is, how you live, the noise you make, how you spit, or what language you use. ... We decide what is right. Never mind what the people think. We know what we have to do which is necessary for the people's survival. Then we set out to persuade people to accept it.

In the minds of the PAP ruling class, if the corporate state is to maximize its profitability, everything needs to remain paternalistically under its control. When it comes to marriage and procreation policy, for instance, a Singaporean man who decides to get married to a non-Singaporean woman will find their marriage plans almost immediately authorized and their future children eligible for citizenship, provided that the wife is highly educated and professionally qualified. On the contrary, if the prospective wife belongs to a lower socioeconomic class, lengthy waiting time is inflicted upon the couple before issuing the marriage authorization (Chua, 1995: 68–69).

In the same spirit, the 1983 Graduate Mothers' Scheme, later abandoned due to its extreme unpopularity, urged highly educated women, supposedly capable of breeding better-performing children, to have more of them in order to improve the overall gene pool of the Singaporean population. Lee Kuan Yew declared that the problem of unmarried female graduates is linked to the problem of a declining birth rate and will affect the quality of future generations. ... If we go on at this rate, we will not be reproducing the kind of society we are in 20 years. It will be a society with a lower level of performance. ... We are born unequal, and we have got to make the best of the lot. ... The more we have of people who can run the economy, the better. (*The Straits Times*, 1986)

A similar eugenic-based measure, this time addressed to lower class women, was the sterilization programme of 1984. This policy granted financial support to low-income and low-educated women willing to be sterilized (Palen, 1986). An analogous measure still exists to this very day though it does not involve sterilization. The Home Ownership Plus Education (HOPE) Scheme makes poor and less educated women eligible for a housing grant of up to $60,000 if they keep their families small. These extreme population planning policies all stem from the belief, held by Lee and the PAP ruling class at large, that without properly "scientific" eugenic policies that promoted breeding among the elite, Singapore would become a "society with a large number of the physically, intellectually and culturally anemic" (Tan, 2003: 415), thus ultimately hurting the economic competitiveness of the Singaporean nation-corporation.

Finally, even issues of public morality are put through the pragmatic-neoliberal sieve. Taboo activities are allowed or forbidden by the PAP regime based on their potential profitability. An emblematic case of this was the authorization of casino gambling. The legalization of casinos in the mid-2000s was met with massive public backlash, especially from conservative and religious organizations. The criticisms levied by these groups, highlighting the negative societal externalities of large-scale gambling, were not much different from the arguments the PAP leaders themselves had offered up until then to justify their reluctance to legalize casinos. However, once the Singaporean government grasped the profit potential of casino resorts in terms of tourism revenues, it changed its mind. In fact, casino legalization soon became an indispensable piece of the city-state's global-city strategy. With little hesitation, moral and social concerns were set aside and priority was given to economic pursuits. The opponents of legalized casino gambling were presented with the hard truth that economic opportunity trumps public opinion (Wee, 2012).

THE SINGAPORE MODEL ABROAD

Singapore's early espousal of neoliberalism has certainly borne good fruit. The virtually unmatched economic development of the city-state, which Lee Kuan Yew (2000) has efficaciously encapsulated in the phrase "from Third World to First", is hard to dispute. In 1965, the income of the average Singaporean stood at US$516 per year, on par with that of the then-average Jordanian or Mexican. In 2020, Singapore's GDP per capita of over US$65,000 came in at seventh position worldwide, ranking between Iceland (sixth) and the United States (eighth) (World Bank, 2020b). Moreover, Singapore's outstanding achievements have been more than just economic ones. As Mahbubani (2015) recalls in an article titled "why Singapore is the world's most successful society",

> We had reduced our infant mortality faster than any other society, going down from 35 per 1,000 live births in 1965 to 10.90 in 1985. … The babies who lived in Singapore went on to enjoy one of the best education systems in the world. The OECD ranked 15-year-old Singaporean children number one in the world in a recent global ranking of "Universal Basic Skills" in mathematics and science. Singapore students also topped the OECD PISA problem-solving test in 2012. … From the Singapore with slums that I grew up in, we now have the highest home ownership of any country in the world, with 90 percent of residents living in homes they own. Even amongst households in the lowest 20 percent of incomes, over 80 percent own their own homes. … Singapore is one of the best places to be born in and to live in. Quite amazingly, a society destined to fail in 1965 has become one of the world's greatest success stories.

Besides being a source of national pride for Singaporeans, the economic success of the Singapore model has inspired many from all over the world. Politicians, economists, and commentators from all across the ideological spectrum have publicly praised the virtues of the Singaporean development experience.

Milton Friedman, Nobel prize-winning conservative economist and free market enthusiast, often pointed to Singapore as a quintessential example of how the pursuit of acute economic freedom is key to a country's development. He once famously said that "if you compare the conditions of people in a place like Singapore with the conditions of people in a place like red China or for that matter Indonesia, you will see that the economic freedom is a very important component of total freedom" (Zarroli, 2015). Former left-of-centre UK Prime Minister Tony Blair was also an enthusiastic fan of the city-state, its strong government, the fertile ground for global business, and its firm grip on society (Faucher-King and Le Galès, 2010: 133). Words of praise also came from former UN Secretary General Kofi Annan, who wrote that the Singaporean development experience "will be of great interest to people of other developing countries and to all those who are interested in their fate" (Lee, 2000, back cover).

In addition to the countless verbal expressions of admiration for the Singapore model, there have been many worldwide attempts to replicate it. From Putin's wish to turn the newly annexed Crimea into a global trade centre like Singapore (Pismennaya, 2014), to Rwanda, which dispatched delegations to the city-state to explore ways to transform itself from a local trading post into a worldwide commercial hub (Chu, 2009), passing through the dream of Indian metropolis Bangalore to become "the Singapore of South India" (Nair, 2005: 124), there are numerous countries that have expressed a wish to emulate the Singapore miracle. Even the UK—of which Singapore was a former colony—has flirted with the post-Brexit possibility of turning into a "Singapore-upon-Thames" (McTague and Guerrera, 2017; Parker et al., 2017).

In a Time of Crisis, a Victim of Its Own (Neoliberal) Success?

The view from inside Singapore seems less laudatory and rather more mixed. In the words of Yeoh Lam Keong, former Chief Economist at Government Investment Corporation (GIC), Singapore's sovereign wealth fund, "on the surface of it, [the Singapore economy] looks astonishingly miraculous. Everybody thinks it's a perfect economy. ... But that's on the surface" (cited in Guest, 2020).

Much like in many other advanced countries over the last ten years, a number of latent social issues, which had lurked in the background for decades, have finally come out into the open. In fact, Singapore is going through a period of socioeconomic and political metamorphosis. Local and global trends are intersecting to bring about a new socio-political environment in the city-state, a "new normal" (Low et al., 2014: 1). This started at the onset of the new millennium and markedly hastened with the 2011 General Election, when the PAP was confronted with its worst electoral performance since independence. The current COVID-19 pandemic is proving a formidable stress test for the Singapore model, combining and synthesizing these multiple crises into a perfect storm.

Income Inequality. The first major challenge to the Singapore model to emerge in recent years is economic inequality and social immobility. Since independence, the PAP government's political legitimacy had not been derived exclusively from electoral democracy, but rather from sustained economic performance. In the last decade or so, the unwritten social contract between government and citizens has been slowly eroding. The prospects of improving one's life chances by means of education and hard work seem to be gradually waning in a society that is shifting from meritocracy to elitism (Guest, 2020; Tan, 2008). As the social elevator slows down, so has the promise of a widespread distribution of the fruits of economic growth. Even though average per capita income has indeed increased over the last decades, the city-state remains one of the most unequal among advanced countries. Wages at the lower end of the income distribution are remarkably low when compared to most other developed economies. And, although there is mounting evidence that progress has indeed been made in stabilizing and even partially redressing economic disparities over the last decade (Peng, 2019), income inequality in Singapore remains worryingly above a Gini coefficient of 0.4, an alert threshold which has been described by experts worldwide as potentially dangerous for social stability if exceeded (Guo, 2016: 232; Tao et al., 2017).

Ever since the 1980s, the logics of globalization, coupled with the PAP's neoliberal policies, have driven an ever-increasing wedge between those high up the income ladder and those at the bottom. After two decades of extensive economic prosperity, in fact, Singapore's rising tide appeared not to be lifting all boats anymore. Singaporean sociologist Ern Ser Tan (2015: 128) argued that:

> From the mid-80s onwards, the Singapore Dream has increasingly come under serious threat not only in the forms of economic fluctuations, stiff global competition and technological changes, but also cost inflation, low fertility and a rapidly ageing population, giving rise to the need to further liberalise the inflow of migrants and foreign labour. All of these processes have contributed in one way or another to the widening income gap. ... There is a concern that the widening income gap ... would act as a dampener on upward social mobility for those on the lower and middle segments

of the social ladder, resulting in class origin largely determining destiny once again.

The PAP regime is certainly not unaware of Singapore's inequality-immobility nexus. In 2018, Senior Minister Tharman Shanmugaratnam publicly declared that "once … that escalator that carries everyone up stops, the problems of inequality and all the problems of me against you, this group against that group, become much sharper" (Kok, 2019). However, the acknowledgement of the problem on the part of the government has not been matched by solutions radical enough to meet the challenge. To be fair, there have been increases in social expenditure directed at individuals and families in the low- and middle-income strata, especially in the COVID-19 national budgets. However, other than "fire-fighting" efforts to mitigate the injuries of the pandemic, more structurally oriented policies that could address longer-term inequality-reducing objectives, have been remarkably tame (Low et al., 2014: X).

In a 2018 report titled "The Commitment to Reducing Inequality Index 2018", Oxfam and Development Finance International placed Singapore in 149th position out of 157 countries in terms of its efforts to tackle economic inequality (Lawson and Martin, 2018). Singapore's disappointing placement among the world's bottom 10 countries is mainly to be attributed to the city-state's inadequacies with respect to tax practices, social spending, and labour protection legislation. Lee Hsien Loong responded:

> that we achieved [economic prosperity] with lower taxes and lower spending than most countries is to Singapore's credit rather than discredit. … We set out to achieve real outcomes for our people – good health, education, jobs and housing – rather than satisfy a collection of ideologically driven indicators. (Yahya, 2018)

However, in spite of the government's counter-narrative efforts, there still remains a widespread perception that Singapore works far better for the wealthy than for the average citizen (Yeo, 2020).

The advent of the COVID-19 crisis has done nothing but exacerbate this trend. As global billionaires amass unprecedented levels of wealth, low-wage workers worldwide are paying the price of the coronavirus pandemic with little social or financial protection (Gneiting et al., 2020).

Singapore is no exception. The city-state's urban poor, the greatly over-looked members of Asia's most affluent society, are now the most severely affected by the crisis. Like never before, COVID-19 appears to have widened the chasm between the affluent and the worst-off in Singapore society (Toh, 2020). As a reaction to the crisis, the government has mobilized an impressive 19% of its GDP to save jobs and support workers and businesses. Yet, in the grand scheme of things, this is unlikely to be even remotely sufficient. In the midst of the crisis, the government's trickle-down approach to state assistance that focused on supporting companies and employers did not always produce benefits that percolated down to all workers equally (Teo and Ng, 2020). In response to what has been dubbed the world's deepest recession since World War II (World Bank, 2020a), a wider, more comprehensive scheme of inequality reduction is necessary.

Migrant Workers. Equally concerning for the future of Singapore is the issue of immigration. The COVID-19 crisis has shed new light on one of Singapore's flagship neoliberal policies, the massive inpouring of cheap migrant labour. Up until late-March, when extensive COVID-19 outbreaks began in migrant worker dormitories, Singapore had been hailed internationally as the "gold standard" for its effective response to the coronavirus pandemic (Griffiths, 2020). Even though the large-scale clusters in the dormitories, which make up over 90% of the total number of cases in Singapore, were initially blamed on the "communal living of migrant workers, suggesting cultural-behavioural roots of the infections" (Dutta, 2020: 14), it soon became clear that the reason behind the surge in migrant worker cases was to be found elsewhere.

In contrast with many mainstream media narratives, the low hygiene standards in migrant worker dormitories that helped rapidly spread the infection among workers were in fact a consequence of the cramped living conditions forced upon them, not a result of their cultural predilection for such a tightly communal living environment. As early as 23 March 2020, well before the infection thoroughly took hold in the dorms, advocacy group Transient Workers Count Too (TWC2) warned in an open letter published in local broadsheet *The Straits Times* that it was virtually impossible for migrants to obey social distancing rules in such a highly crammed setting and that, without proper intervention, a public health catastrophe in the dormitories was inevitable (TWC2, 2020). The government appeared to have ignored these warnings. Soon enough, while it was focusing its world-class coronavirus response on mainstream society or "the community", an explosion of cases occurred in the overlooked migrant dormitories.

The blatantly differential treatment of Singapore citizens and permanent residents at one end and migrant workers at the other is reflected in, among other things, the government's daily reporting of inflection rates that presented the two groups separately (Han, 2020). Such institutionalized discrimination points to the all-too-familiar neoliberal conception of foreign workers as mere economic tools for Singapore's prosperity. Necessary yet undesirable, migrant workers are hidden from the community's sight and, in a way that is reminiscent of Lefebvre's politics of space (1991), confined to peripheral dormitories, a precise urban space compatible with the role they play within the Singaporean capitalist society. However, this neoliberal strategy of segregation and neglect is what ultimately let down Singapore's much admired coronavirus response, threatening the country's overall well-being. To quote Alex Au, vice-president of TWC2,

> The problem here is Singapore's whole economic model, our prosperity, is really built on the assumption or expectation of cheap labour … [COVID-19 has shown] us that cheap is a temporary thing. There will be hidden costs that will erupt when you do not expect it. (Quoted in Ng, 2020)

COURSE CORRECTION: TOWARDS A MORE INCLUSIVE CITY-STATE?

Most of these problems, from economic inequality to the poor treatment of migrant workers, have been afflicting Singapore society well before the beginning of the pandemic. As an unwanted catalyst, however, the coronavirus crisis has had the unique capacity to conflate all of them into one massive predicament. Yet this also provides Singapore with an opportunity to meet the challenge head-on. Some members of the most boldly progressive sections of the PAP have shown they are ready to seize it. In the words of Tharman Shanmugaratnam (2020),

> It did not begin with the pandemic. Social divisions were already growing …. But they are now getting even wider. Job and income losses have hit some groups much harder than others. Children without well-off parents are falling behind …. All this is sharpening feelings of helplessness, and the

sense that the system is stacked against those who are already disadvantaged. And it is bringing long-standing perceptions of racial injustice to a boiling point. ... The economic dangers we now face compel us to fortify our society.

At a time when the coronavirus has the potential to "spell the end of the neoliberal era" (Lent, 2020), it is only reasonable that Singapore, having subscribed so fully and uncritically to the neoliberal dogma, would also go through a hard time. By virtue of its "evolutionary" nature (Schumpeter, 1962: 82), and as it has always done, capitalism will most likely survive the end of the neoliberal age and, by incorporating elements of social protection into its neoliberal frame, will reinvent itself to suit what will come next.

Singapore should do the same. If it were truly pragmatic, the PAP government should also strive to really rethink itself and the city-state in this era of epochal change.

REFERENCES

Au Yong, J. (2009, October 20). MM Lee: Social Divide Inevitable. *The Straits Times*, p. A8. https://www.smu.edu.sg/sites/default/files/smu/news_r oom/smu_in_the_news/2009/sources/ST_20091020_3.pdf. Accessed 9 October 2020.

Birch, K., & Mykhnenko, V. (2009). Varieties of Neoliberalism? Restructuring in Large Industrially Dependent Regions Across Western And Eastern Europe. *Journal of Economic Geography*, 9(3), 355–380.

Bloom, P. (2016). *Authoritarian Capitalism in the Age of Globalization*. Cheltenham: Edward Elgar Press.

Brown, D. (1998). Globalisation, Ethnicity and the Nation-State: The Case of Singapore. *Australian Journal of International Affairs*, 52(1), 35–46.

Chang, J. Y. (2019). Conscripting the Audience: Singapore's Successful Securitisation of Vulnerability. In S. H. Ho & G. Ong-Webb (Eds.), *National Service in Singapore* (pp. 83–103). Singapore: World Scientific Publishing.

Chew, P. G. L. (2000). Islands and National Identity: The Metaphors of Singapore. *International Journal of the Sociology of Language*, 143(1), 121–137.

Chu, J. (2009, January 4). Rwanda Rising: A New Model of Economic Development. *Fast Company*. https://www.fastcompany.com/1208900/rwanda-ris ing-new-model-economic-development. Accessed 11 October 2020.

Chua, B. H. (1995). *Communitarian Ideology and Democracy in Singapore*. London: Routledge.

Chua, B. H. (2019). Singapore from Social Democracy to Communitarianism. In W. Reese-Schäfer (Ed.), *Handbuch Kommunitarismus* (pp. 643–662). Wiesbaden: Springer VS.

Cooper Ramo, J. (2004). *The Beijing Consensus: Notes on the New Physics of Chinese Power*. London: Foreign Policy Centre.

Dent, C. M. (2001). Singapore's Foreign Economic Policy: The Pursuit of Economic Security. *Contemporary Southeast Asia*, 23(1), 1–23.

Dutta, M. J. (2020). COVID-19, Authoritarian Neoliberalism, and Precarious Migrant Work in Singapore: Structural Violence and Communicative Inequality. *Frontiers in Communication*, 5(58), 1–18.

Faucher-King, F., & Le Galès, P. (2010). *The New Labour Experiment: Change and Reform Under Blair and Brown*. Stanford, California: Stanford University Press.

Florida, R. L. (2002). *The Rise of the Creative Class: And How It's Transforming Work, Leisure, Community and Everyday Life*. New York, NY: Basic Books.

Garfinkle, A. (2020, January 24). Overdoing It, with Chinese Characteristics. *The American Interest*. https://www.the-american-interest.com/2020/01/24/overdoing-it-with-chinese-characteristics/. Accessed 13 November 2020.

Gibson, W. (1993, September-October). Disneyland with the Death Penalty. *Wired*. https://www.wired.com/1993/04/gibson-2/. Accessed 8 October 2020.

Gneiting, U., Lusiani, N., & Tamir, I. (2020). *Power, Profits and the Pandemic*. Oxfam Briefing Paper. https://www.oxfam.org/en/research/power-profits-and-pandemic. Accessed 12 October 2020.

Goh, C. T. (2002, August 18). *National Day Rally 2002*. University Cultural Centre at National University of Singapore, Singapore. https://www.nas.gov.sg/archivesonline/data/pdfdoc/2002081805.htm. Accessed 9 October 2020.

Griffiths, J. (2020, April 19). Singapore Had a Model Coronavirus Response, Then Cases Spiked. What Happened? *CNN*. https://edition.cnn.com/2020/04/18/asia/singapore-coronavirus-response-intl-hnk/index.html. Accessed 12 October 2020.

Guest, P. (2020, January 22). Is Singapore's 'Perfect' Economy Coming Apart? *Nikkei Asia*. https://asia.nikkei.com/Spotlight/The-Big-Story/Is-Singapore-s-perfect-economy-coming-apart. Accessed 11 October 2020.

Guo, Y. (2016). *Handbook on Class and Social Stratification in China*. Edward Elgar Publishing.

Guo, Y., & Woo, J. J. (2013, September 20). The Secrets to Small State Survival. *The Straits Times*. https://www.straitstimes.com/singapore/the-secrets-to-small-state-survival. Accessed 24 September 2020.

Han, J., & Seng, L. T. (2014, July 4). Industrial Relations (Amendment) Act. National Library Board. https://eresources.nlb.gov.sg/infopedia/art icles/SIP_2014-07-07_133856.html. Accessed 9 October 2020.

Han, K. (2020, May 6). Singapore Is Trying to Forget Migrant Workers Are People. *Foreign Policy.* https://foreignpolicy.com/2020/05/06/singapore-coronavirus-~pandemic-migrant-workers/. Accessed 15 October 2020.

Harvey, D. (2005). *A Brief History of Neoliberalism.* Oxford: Oxford University Press.

Heng, Y. (2013). A Global City in an Age of Global Risks: Singapore's Evolving Discourse on Vulnerability. *Contemporary Southeast Asia,* 35(3), 423–446.

Heracleous, L. (2001). State Ownership, Privatization and Performance in Singapore: An Exploratory Study from a Strategic Management Perspective. *Asia Pacific Journal of Management,* 18, 69–81.

Hill, M. & Varone, F. (2017). *The Public Policy Process* (7th ed.). London and New York: Routledge.

Ho, P. (2018). *The Challenges of Governance in a Complex World.* Singapore: World Scientific Publishing.

Hooi, A. (2004, December 24). Let Market Decide Maid Wages, Agencies Told. *The Straits Times,* p. 4. https://advance-lexis-com.libproxy1.nus.edu. sg/api/document?collection=news&id=urn:contentItem:4F38-8NX0-0058-X48M-00000-00&context=1516831. Accessed 9 October 2020.

Kok, X. (2019, November 18). If Singapore Is So Wealthy, Why Do Its Citizens Feel Stuck? *South China Morning Post.* https://www.scmp.com/week-asia/economics/article/3037984/if-singapore-so-wealthy-why-do-its-citizens-feel-stuck. Accessed 12 October 2020.

Kraar, L. (1974, July). Singapore, the Country Run Like a Corporation. *Fortune.* https://fortune.com/2015/03/23/singapore-leekuanyew-corporation-1974/. Accessed 5 October 2020.

Lawson, M., & Martin, M. (2018). *The Commitment to Reducing Inequality Index 2018.* Oxfam and Development Finance International report. https://oxfamilibrary.openrepository.com/bitstream/handle/10546/620553/rr-commitment-reducing-inequality-index-2018-091018-en.pdf. Accessed 12 October 2020.

Lee, H. L. (2007, August 19). *National Day Rally 2007.* University Cultural Centre at National University of Singapore, Singapore. https://www.pmo. gov.sg/Newsroom/pm-lee-hsien-loongs-national-day-rally-speech-2007-english. Accessed 9 October 2020.

Lee, H. L. (2010, August 29). *National Day Rally 2010.* University Cultural Centre at National University of Singapore, Singapore. https://www.pmo.gov.sg/Newsroom/prime-minister-lee-hsien-loongs-national-day-rally-2010-speech-english. Accessed 8 October 2020.

Lee, K. Y. (1957). *Parliamentary Speech*. Singapore Legislative Assembly, Debates III, no. 20 (5 March), col. 1,471.

Lee, K. Y. (1986, August 17). *National Day Rally 1986*. Kallang Theatre, Singapore. https://www.nas.gov.sg/archivesonline/audiovisual_rec ords/record-details/48aabfb1-1164-11e3-83d5-0050568939ad. Accessed 10 October 2020.

Lee, K. Y. (2000). *From Third World to First: The Singapore Story, 1965-2000: Singapore and the Asian Economic Boom*. New York: HarperCollins Publishers.

Lee, K. Y. (2003, February 18). *Senior Minister Lee Kuan Yew's Q&A session at NTU Students' Union (9th Ministerial Forum)*. Nanyang Auditorium at Nanyang Technological University, Singapore. https://www.nas.gov.sg/arc hivesonline/data/pdfdoc/2003021806.htm. Accessed 9 October 2020.

Lee, K. Y. (2009, April 9). *Speech by Mr. Lee Kuan Yew, Minister Mentor, at the S. Rajaratnam Lecture*. Shangri-La Hotel, Singapore. https://www.pmo. gov.sg/Newsroom/speech-mr-lee-kuan-yew-minister-mentor-s-rajaratnam-lec ture-09-april-2009-530-pm-shangri. Accessed 1 October 2020.

Lefebvre, H. (1991). *The Production of Space*. Blackwell: Oxford.

Leggett, C. J. (2005). *Strategic Choice and the Transformations of Singapore's Industrial Relations*. Thesis (PhD Doctorate). Griffith Business School, Queensland, Australia. https://research-repository.griffith.edu.au/bitstream/handle/10072/365411/02Whole.pdf?sequence=1. Accessed 8 May 2021.

Lent, J. (2020, April 12). Coronavirus Spells the End of the Neoliberal Era. What's Next? *openDemocracy*. https://www.opendemocracy.net/en/tra nsformation/coronavirus-spells-the-end-of-the-neoliberal-era-whats-next/. Accessed 13 October 2020.

LePoer, B. L. (1989). *Singapore: A Country Study*. Washington, DC: Federal Research Division, Library of Congress. https://tile.loc.gov/storage-ser vices/master/frd/frdcstdy/si/singaporecountry00lepo/singaporecountry00 lepo_djvu.txt. Accessed 9 October 2020.

Letelier, O. (1976). *Chile, Economic Freedom and Political Repression*. Nottingham: Bertrand Russell Peace Foundation.

Liow, E. D. (2012). The Neoliberal-Developmental State: Singapore as Case Study. *Critical Sociology*, 38(2), 241–264.

Low, D., Vadaketh, S. T., Lim, L., & Thum, P. (2014). *Hard Choices: Challenging the Singapore Consensus*. Singapore: NUS Press.

Low, L. (2002a). Rethinking Singapore Inc. and GLCs. *Southeast Asian Affairs*, 282–302.

Low, L. (2002b). The Political Economy of Migrant Worker Policy in Singapore. *Asia Pacific Business Review*, 8(4), 95–118.

Luther, H. (1979). The Repression of Labour Protest in Singapore: Unique Case or Future Model? *Development and Change*, 10(2), 287-299.

Magcamit, M. I. (2015). Trading in Paranoia: Exploring Singapore's Security-Trade Linkages in the Twenty-first Century. *Asian Journal of Political Science*, 23(2), 184–206.

Mahbubani, K. (2010). Results Matter: Pragmatism Prevails in Asia. *Global Asia*, 5(1), 37–42.

Mahbubani, K. (2015, April 8). Why Singapore Is the World's Most Successful Society. *HuffPost*. https://www.huffpost.com/entry/singapore-world-succes sful-society_b_7934988. Accessed 5 October 2020.

McTague, T., & Guerrera, F. (2017, January 18). Britain's Singapore Threat. *POLITICO Europe*. https://www.politico.eu/article/britains-singapore-thr eat-philip-hammond-may-brexit/. Accessed 11 October 2020.

Nair, J. (2005). *The Promise of the Metropolis: Bangalore's Twentieth Century*. Oxford: Oxford University Press.

Naruse, C. N., & Gui, W. (2016). Singapore and the Intersections of Neoliberal Globalization and Postcoloniality. *Interventions*, 18(4), 473-482.

Ng, E. (2020, April 10). Low-Paid Migrant Workers Bear the Worst of Singapore's Second COVID-19 Wave. *People's World*. https://www.peoplesworld. org/article/low-paid-migrant-workers-bear-the-worst-of-singapores-second-covid-19-wave/. Accessed 12 October 2020.

Ortmann, S. (2012). The 'Beijing Consensus' and the 'Singapore Model': Unmasking the Myth of an Alternative Authoritarian State-Capitalist Model. *Journal of Chinese Economic and Business Studies*, 10(4), 337–359.

Palen, J. J. (1986). Fertility and Eugenics: Singapore's Population Policies. *Population Research and Policy Review*, 5(1), 3–14.

Parker, G., Ford, J., & Barker, A. (2017, January 19). Is Theresa May's Brexit Plan B an Elaborate Bluff? *Financial Times*. https://www.ft.com/content/ 3501446a-de36-11e6-86ac-f253db7791c6. Accessed 11 October 2020.

Peng, N. (2019). Inequality and the Social Compact in Singapore: Macro Trends Versus Lived Realities. *Journal of Southeast Asian Economies*, 36(3), 355–379.

Peng, N., & Phang, S. Y. (2018). Singapore's Economic Development: Pro- or Anti-Washington Consensus? *Economic and Political Studies*, 6(1), 30–52.

Pismennaya, E. (2014, May 22). Putin's Singapore Dream Costs Crimea Banks and Burgers. *Bloomberg*. https://www.bloomberg.com/news/articles/2014-05-22/putin-s-singapore-dream-costs-crimea-banks-and-burgers. Accessed 11 October 2020.

Rajaratnam, S. (1972, February 6). *Singapore: Global City*. Text of an Address to the Singapore Press Club. Ministry of Culture, Singapore. https://www. nas.gov.sg/archivesonline/data/pdfdoc/PressR19720206a.pdf. Accessed 2 October 2020.

Rutland, P. (2013). Neoliberalism and the Russian transition. *Review of International Political Economy*, 20(2), 332–362.

Schumpeter, J. A. (1962). *Capitalism, Socialism and Democracy.* New York: Harper Torchbooks.

Schwartz, P. (2010, January 14). Singapore: The Apple of Nations. *Ethos*, Issue 7. https://www.csc.gov.sg/articles/singapore-the-apple-of-nations. Accessed 8 October 2020.

Shanmugaratnam, T. (2020, June 17). *A Stronger and More Cohesive Society.* National Broadcast. https://www.gov.sg/article/senior-minister-tharman-sha nmugaratnam-a-stronger-and-more-cohesive-society. Accessed 12 October 2020.

Singh, R. S. (2019). In the Company of Citizens: The Rhetorical Contours of Singapore's Neoliberalism. *Communication and Critical/Cultural Studies*, 16(3), 161–177.

Tan, E. S. (2015). *Social Mobility in Singapore.* In D. Chan (Ed.), *50 Years of Social Issues in Singapore* (pp. 119–132). Singapore: World Scientific.

Tan, K. P. (2001). Civic Society and the New Economy in Patriarchal Singapore: Emasculating the Political, Feminizing the Public. *Crossroads: An Interdisciplinary Journal of Southeast Asian Studies*, 15(2), 95–122.

Tan, K. P. (2003). Sexing Up Singapore. *International Journal of Cultural Studies*, 6(4), 403–423.

Tan, K. P. (2008). Meritocracy and Elitism in a Global City: Ideological Shifts in Singapore. *International Political Science Review*, 29(1): 7–27.

Tan, K. P. (2017). *Governing Global-City Singapore: Legacies and Futures After Lee Kuan Yew.* London: Routledge.

Tao, Y., Wu, X., & Li, C. (2017, September 26). *Rawls' Fairness, Income Distribution and Alarming Level of Gini Coefficient.* Economics Discussion Papers, No 2017–67, Kiel Institute for the World Economy. https://arxiv.org/ftp/arxiv/papers/1409/1409.3979.pdf. Accessed 9 May 2021.

Tay, T. F. (2019, February 12). Parliament: SingPost Not the Only Mail Operator. *The Straits Times.* https://www.straitstimes.com/singapore/singpost-not-the-only-mail-operator. Accessed 9 May 2021.

Teo, S. (2014). State of the Arts: Government, National Identity, and the Arts in Singapore. *Undergraduate Humanities Forum 2013–2014: Violence*, 1. https://repository.upenn.edu/cgi/viewcontent.cgi?article=1010&context=uhf_2014. Accessed 13 November 2020.

Teo, Y. Y., & Ng, K. H. (2020, March 17). Crisis Is Exactly the Time to Make Structural Changes to Address Poverty and Inequality. *Academia.SG.* https://www.academia.sg/academic-views/crisis-is-exactly-the-time-to-make-structural-changes-to-address-poverty-and-inequality/. Accessed 12 October 2020.

The Straits Times. (1986, August 18). More Graduate Men Marrying Graduate Women. *The Straits Times*, p. 8. https://eresources.nlb.gov.sg/newspapers/Digitised/Article/straitstimes19860818-1.2.18.1?ST=1&AT=search&k=18%20august%201986&QT=18,august,1986&oref=article. Accessed 10 October 2020.

The Straits Times. (1995, May 6). New Code to Boost the 'Service' in Civil Service. *The Straits Times*, p. 2. https://eresources.nlb.gov.sg/newspapers/Digitised/Article/straitstimes19950506-1.2.76.3.1. Accessed 7 May 2021.

Toh, E. M. (2020, April 8). Pushed Down a Rung. *Southeast Asia Globe*. https://southeastasiaglobe.com/singapore-urban-poor-covid/. Accessed 12 October 2020.

TWC2. (2020, March 23). *Straits Times Forum: Employers' Practices Leave Foreign Workers Vulnerable to Infection*. https://twc2.org.sg/2020/03/23/straits-times-forumemployers-practices-leave-foreign-workers-vulnerable-to-inf ection/. Accessed 13 November 2020.

Wang, J. (2012). The Developmental State in the Global Hegemony of Neoliberalism: A New Strategy for Public Housing in Singapore. *Cities*, 29(6), 369–378.

Wee, L. (2012). Neoliberalism and the Regulation of Consumers: Legalizing Casinos in Singapore. *Critical Discourse Studies*, 9(1), 15–27.

World Bank. (2020a). *Global Economic Prospects*. Washington, DC: World Bank. https://openknowledge.worldbank.org/handle/10986/33748. Accessed 17 November 2020.

World Bank, World Development Indicators. (2020b). *GDP per capita (current US$)* [Data file]. https://data.worldbank.org/indicator/NY.GDP.PCAP.CD. Accessed 11 October 2020.

Yahya, Y. (2018, October 9). Singapore Refutes Oxfam Report on Its Performance in Tackling Inequality. *The Straits Times*. https://www.straitstimes.com/singapore/singapore-refutes-oxfam-report-on-its-performance-in-tackling-inequality. Accessed 12 October 2020.

Yeo, J. (2020, January 5). S'pore Has 207,000 Millionaires in 2019, but over 700,000 Have Less Than S$13,500 to Their Name. *Mothership.SG*. https://mothership.sg/2020/01/singapore-millionaires/#:~:text=Singapore%20saw%20a%20rise%20in,S%241.35%20million)%20in%20wealth. Accessed 12 October 2020.

Zarroli, J. (2015, March 29). How Singapore Became One of the Richest Places on Earth. *NPR*. https://www.npr.org/2015/03/29/395811510/how-singapore-became-one-of-the-richest-places-on-earth. Accessed 15 October 2020.

Zohlnhöfer, R., Engler, F., & Dümig, K. (2018). The Retreat of the Interventionist State in Advanced Democracies. *British Journal of Political Science*, 48(2), 535–562.

CHAPTER 3

Public Health Legacies: Tuberculosis, HIV/AIDS, and SARS in Singapore

Hongwu Lyu and Aymeric Vo Quang

Abstract Tuberculosis, HIV/AIDS, and Severe Acute Respiratory Syndrome (SARS) are historically significant cases of infectious disease outbreaks that have posed economic, social, reputational, and moral challenges to Singapore and its much-vaunted model. Until only in recent years, Singapore's neoliberal public health system—focused on efficiency and optimal allocation—had neglected HIV/AIDS and thus the segments of society often associated with it. This neglect had been heightened by prevailing social stigmas and stereotypes. This may shed some light on the COVID-19 pandemic, which elicited rapid, responsive, robust, and inclusive government action where mainstream Singaporean community was concerned, but at the same time failed to recognize and deal

H. Lyu (✉)
Double Master Degree in Public Policy and European Affairs, National University of Singapore and Sciences Po (2021), Hangzhou, China
e-mail: e0404067@u.nus.edu; hongwu.lyu@sciencespo.fr

A. Vo Quang
Double Master Degree in Public Policy and European Affairs, National University of Singapore and Sciences Po (2021), Versailles, France
e-mail: e0404073@u.nus.edu; aymeric.voquang@sciencespo.fr

© The Author(s), under exclusive license to Springer Nature Singapore Pte Ltd. 2022
K. P. Tan (ed.), *Singapore's First Year of COVID-19*,
https://doi.org/10.1007/978-981-19-0368-7_3

53

with the marginalized and possibly stigmatized segments of society, such as migrant workers, whose badly infected dormitories became an international spectacle of crisis and social injustice. COVID-19 resembled tuberculosis and HIV/AIDS in terms of social stigmatization and even moral panic over the unhealthy elements in society. This resulted in the othering of—and disproportionate concern and hostility towards—teenage "spitters" who threatened to spread tuberculosis through their "defiant" behaviour, homosexuals who threatened to spread HIV/AIDS through their "immoral" behaviour and migrant workers in dormitories who were the foreign bringers of disease. The SARS crisis in 2003 was a "wake-up call" for a less-than-prepared Singapore. A subsequently more proactive government learnt key lessons from the crisis, which were systematically institutionalized in readiness for the next infectious disease outbreak.

Keywords Public health · Infectious diseases · Tuberculosis · HIV/AIDS · SARS · Stigmatization · Moral panic

In October 1819, only nine months after its founding as a British trading post, Singapore was confronted with its first epidemic. Cholera had made its appearance at another nearby British settlement, Penang and was to spread through most of the Malay Peninsula. Anticipating a southward spread, Singapore's colonial authorities were quick to dispatch medication and implement quarantine measures that successfully protected the island. The very first recorded instance of forced quarantine in Singapore occurred in June 1821 when a cholera-stricken Austrian ship, the *Caroline Augustus*, arrived from Batavia (today's Jakarta) with afflicted sailors. Mindful of the safety of residents in Singapore who had been relatively untouched by cholera, Major-General William Farquhar, British Resident and Commandant of the colony, did not allow the ship to land. He did however let the convalescents get medical assistance at Sandy Point, at the tip of the neighbourhood known today as Tanjong Rhu (Tan, 2020; Lee, 1973). While the cholera epidemic did not establish itself in Singapore at that point in time, it repeatedly threatened the settlement throughout the nineteenth century (in 1841, 1851, 1873, 1895, and 1902), pushing the British colonial administration to improve the city's healthcare and sanitation system.

In 1957, an influenza epidemic arrived in Singapore. Dubbed the "Asian Flu", it had passed through Hong Kong, another globally connected city, to Singapore, before becoming an international pandemic affecting Taiwan, India, the United Kingdom, and the United States. In 2003, there was an outbreak of Severe Acute Respiratory Syndrome (SARS). It was first detected in Foshan, quickly spread to Guangzhou City, another regional trading hub, then to Hong Kong, and then to the rest of the world. It reached Singapore within weeks of its appearance in the southern part of the People's Republic of China (Lee et al., 2007).

From the very beginning of its modern history in 1819, Singapore has been vulnerable to epidemics because of its strategic location along major trade routes between Australasia and Europe. Its vulnerability has not been limited only to regional and tropical diseases such as malaria, dengue fever, and melioidosis, as well as more recent ones like the Nipah virus, H1N1, and H5N1 influenza (Thomas et al., 2016; Lim, 2012; Lee et al., 2007). Today's Singapore is a neoliberal global city, a major transport hub, supported by vast flows of tourists and working immigrants. Standing in a confluence of global pathogen movements, Singapore is a "key node" in the spread of infectious disease. New diseases are easily transported from one city to another, and Singapore is particularly vulnerable as it is an essential link in the global chain (Renia and Ng, 2014). According to Thomas et al. (2016: 41), professors at the National University of Singapore's Saw Swee Hock School of Public Health:

> Cities such as Singapore are key nodes in infectious disease as they are hubs for national, regional, and global spread; bridge human and animal ecosystems; and are hubs for globalisation processes: changing social, economic, and cultural structures, increasing personal mobility, cross-boundary integration, and extended and evolving social networks — all driving forces of disease dynamics.

Singapore survives and prospers through its openness, participation, and integration in the global economy. Yet, globalization and urbanization have accelerated the spread of contagious diseases and made Singapore more vulnerable to human pandemics. This results in a paradoxical situation where neoliberal globalization has put Singapore's economy and public health at odds with each other.

A NEOLIBERAL PUBLIC HEALTH SYSTEM

Rapid socio-economic development has brought about significant improvements in infrastructure and health services. These improvements, in turn, have resulted in significantly better health indicators in the city-state. From 1960 to 2019, life expectancy at birth increased from 65.6 to 83.6 years. Infant mortality decreased from 34.9 per 1,000 live births in 1960 to 1.7 per 1,000 live births in 2019, one of the lowest in the world (DOS, 2020; World Bank, 2019; Thomas et al., 2016). Underlying this spectacular socio-economic development especially since the mid-1980s is neoliberal globalization, which has also, in many ways, shaped the public health system.

In 1960, the newly elected People's Action Party (PAP) government introduced a user fee of 50 cents per attendance at government outpatient clinics. Even though the actual cost recovery was negligible, the introduction of a principle of "co-payment" foreshadowed the post-independence government mindset on healthcare (Lim, 2012). The British had left behind a system of government-run hospitals and primary care clinics that was funded by general taxation. In the 1970s, healthcare expenditures increased by four times, due to a significant rise in hospital admissions. Fearing that citizens might be overusing medication and taking subsidized healthcare for granted, the government shifted the model towards a revised financing system based upon "shared responsibility". The 1983 National Health Plan (NHP) presented a model funded through government subsidies and co-payments by patients, aiming at striking a right balance between sustainability and affordability.

Singapore embarked on a "corporatization" of its public health services in the 1980s. Indeed, the Ministry of Health (MOH) drew on the examples of other neoliberal countries undergoing similar reforms, namely the United States under Ronald Reagan and the United Kingdom under Margaret Thatcher. The model was based on the premise that competition among corporatized entities—known as "restructured hospitals"—would result in a more efficient, responsive, and innovative delivery of health services. For its part, MOH could focus on policy formulation and regulation (Quah and Siong, 2016; Thomas et al., 2016; Lim, 2012). In response to growing public concerns, the MOH had to provide reassurance that the restructured hospitals would still retain the essence of the public service mission and offer subsidized rates for the lower-income groups. In 1993, the government committed itself to a humane guarantee that "no Singaporean will ever be denied needed health care because of lack of funds" (Lim, 1998: 20).

The subsequent years have seen the government continuously attempting to strike an appropriate balance between corporatization of public services and the provision of affordable and good quality healthcare for all Singaporeans:

> The organization of Singapore's public healthcare system has evolved over the years as MOH seeks, on one hand, to find an optimal organization and governance structure to drive productivity, innovation, and cost-effective, value-based care provision; and on the other, ensuring that public sector healthcare institutions stay true to their public mission of providing quality care to all Singaporeans. (Quah and Siong, 2016: 71)

"Shared responsibility" became the central principle underpinning the whole system. It refers to the commitment of the government to continue to subsidize and make healthcare affordable while Singaporeans needed to be responsible for paying their share. Against this backdrop, three general schemes were created, also known as the "3M system". MediSave was set up in 1984 as a national and mandatory medical savings plan that supports Singaporeans and their immediate family members in their medical expenses. As a supplement, MediShield was launched in 1990. This insurance plan aims at supporting the high costs of serious illness treatment and long-term hospitalization. In 1993, MediFund was established as an endowment fund to help poor Singaporeans pay for their remaining medical bills after using the two other schemes. These schemes encourage Singaporeans to be responsible for their own health by saving for medical expenses (Thomas et al., 2016). Patients were required to pay a portion of their medical expenditure and expected to pay more when they demanded better services.

Healthcare in Singapore is viewed as a consumption activity that should not be offered as a free lunch. In fact, the government has been cautious to stay away from what it considers to be "welfarism", or unlimited provision of public health services that it deems "not viable as it breeds dependency on the government" (MOE, 2011). While health and institutional support remain available to all, state funding is a measure of last resort (Lim, 2012). In 2013, the Minister for Health Gan Kim Yong declared: "Our public healthcare institutions must have a public mission with corporate discipline, and not act as if you have a corporate mission with public sector discipline!" (Quah and Siong, 2016, p. 72).

How does the neoliberalization of the public health system, pursued in the name of efficiency, apply when it comes to dealing with infectious diseases? Michael Barr, a regular commentator on the Singaporean political system, has shown that Singapore's healthcare is beset by contradictions and limitations, far from the officially published narrative of a rational, objective, and technocratic system (Barr, 2020). This is especially revealed in the case of AIDS. Since the end of 2015, the newly introduced MediShield Life has covered People Living with HIV/AIDS (PLWHA). HIV antiretroviral drugs, which get PLWHA to an undetectable viral load, preventing in turn onward transmission, have become more accessible. From September 2020 onwards, 16 antiretroviral drugs have been added to the list of subsidized drugs, under two of its schemes known as the Standard Drug List and the Medication Assistance Fund, a scheme to help patients pay for expensive drugs used for specific medical conditions. All subsidized patients living with HIV can receive either a 50% or 75% subsidy when they buy any of the 16 drugs on the list (Lim, 2020; Chong, 2020a).

But it has taken a long time to get to this stage. The first case of HIV infection in Singapore was detected in 1985. In the early 2000s, the numbers of HIV positive people in Singapore differed vastly according to different sources. While the MOH reported 2,508 PLWHA in June 2005, the UNAIDS programme estimated 12,000 HIV-positive people in Singapore as early as 2001 (MOH, 2005; AFP, 2001). In this period, the Singapore government's pragmatic approach to public health resulted in a single-sided approach to AIDS management that emphasized the importance of preventive measures through AIDS education while downplaying restorative healthcare like subsidizing antiretrovirals or funding research in infectious and parasitic diseases (IPDs). Up till then, no government funds had been specifically allocated for AIDS (Ong and Yeoh, 2006).

This led to a paradoxical situation in which Singapore, while "comparable in many ways to developed countries in terms of its advanced medical technology and services", was viewed as "a Third World country for HIV victims" (Ong and Yeoh, 2006: 190; AFP, 2001). In response to these critics and the appeals from some members of the public and non-government organization Action of AIDS (AfA) for subsidization of expensive antiretrovirals, the government invoked the notion of "optimal" allocation. In its view, HIV/AIDS was not among the top killers in Singapore, unlike cancer, diabetes, heart disease, or stroke. As well, antiretrovirals were "experimental" rather than "effective" drugs enabling recovery (Ong and Yeoh, 2006).

Therefore, while HIV numbers were increasing in Singapore, PLWHA had to bear the full costs of expensive antiretrovirals. They could withdraw up to $550 a month on their MediSave account, provided they had sufficient funds. In the early 2000s, antiretrovirals would cost from $1,200 to $1,500 a month, an amount well beyond the MediSave spending cap. The cost of antiretrovirals in Singapore was so high—in fact, the highest in the region – that some patients have been going to Thailand to buy cheaper drugs or have skipped medication altogether (AFP, 2001). According to AfA, in 2001, more than 70% of PLWHA in Singapore were not able to afford any form of antiretrovirals, and fewer than 10% were on optimum treatment (Ong and Yeoh, 2006; AFP, 2001). In short, most of PLWHA were deprived of proper treatment because they had to pay for their medical expenses from their own pockets. In the name of efficiency and optimal allocation, the neoliberal health system de-prioritized HIV-positive patients.

At first glance, both the AIDS epidemic and the current COVID-19 pandemic have been dealt with rather differently. Extraordinary government resources have been deployed in the case of COVID-19, challenging the notion of optimal allocation as resources were directed to all Singaporeans and migrant workers. The government has paid the hospital bills of COVID-19 patients who are citizens, permanent residents, and long-term pass holders (Ching, 2020). Medical teams have been sent to migrant worker facilities to triage and actively test for COVID-19 infection. The migrant workers who tested positive have been admitted for free-of-charge treatment. Those who are clinically stable have received medical care in repurposed facilities. Government subsidies have even been granted to employers so they could continue paying wages throughout the crisis (Goh et al., 2020; Iau, 2020).

Beneath the surface, however, the neoliberal model is a model of exclusion. The pandemic highlighted the enduring factors of poor health among migrant workers in Singapore, including their "crammed living environments incompatible with social distancing, language barriers resulting in discriminate care and limited access to health information, an aversion to seeking medical treatment when symptomatic due to fear of losing jobs or wages, and expensive ambulatory healthcare not covered by existing insurance" (Goh et al., 2020: 1). In short, COVID-19 has elicited a rapid and inclusive response from the government, as it posed a serious threat to the broader community. Yet, the pandemic also revealed the migrants' poor living conditions upon which an exploitative neoliberal model rests.

The optimal allocation of treatment, resulting in the side-lining of PLWHA and, at least initially, migrant workers, has not been simply a product of neoliberal trends. It also has to do with the stigmatization surrounding specific infectious diseases and the people most associated with them.

Moral Panics, Stigmatization, and Threat Perception

The topic of infectious disease is by nature an emotional one. Infectious diseases are distressing as they directly endanger one's life and are perceived as threatening the community as a whole. The gap between the real and the perceived threat can be gauged by the extent of "moral panic" surrounding the outbreak of an infectious disease.

In a moral panic, outrage—and not just simple fear—is widely expressed over a perceived deviant behaviour. It involves stigmatization and the construction of "folk devils", which are highly stylized images of despised and marginalized people, such as ethnic groups, migrant workers, people with HIV/AIDS, and homosexuals. Folk devils represent "all that 'we' some apparently homogenous majority group of good, clean-living, *healthy*, law-abiding folks, are not" (Muzzatti, 2005: 120).

As Michel Foucault (1980) has shown, health is one of the essential objectives of political power and a social condition necessary to ensure order. Therefore, any threat to it must be constrained, whether it be a disease or the carriers of the disease themselves. As a precondition to re-establishing order, a threatening illness and its sufferers often take on the qualities of the folk devil. They are repeatedly stigmatized, enabling the authorities to deal firmly and often forcefully with a tangible and highly visible threat. This reinforces society's perception of the sufferer as a "deviant" (Muzzatti, 2005; Foucault, 1980).

This stigma attached to infectious disease and the sufferers can be traced back to colonial times. They tend to provoke moral panic and social stigma according to the nature and "infectiousness" of the disease, the way it is transmitted, and the type of population at risk of being infected. In the late-nineteenth century, colonial officials and doctors classified tuberculosis (TB) under "constitutional diseases" and as a "fever". Already at that time, social stigma against the disease deterred working-class Chinese sufferers from visiting the hospital. In 1927, social stigma fuelled strong opposition against the building of a sanatorium in Pasir Panjang. "The opposition forced the government to abandon the project and instead consider building the sanatorium at the Trafalgar rubber estate in the distant northeast of Singapore, where new premises for the leprosarium and mental hospital were being planned" (Loh and Hsu, 2020: 54). In the 1940s, the colonial government noticed "wild statements and speculations" circulating among the general population regarding the incidence of TB, resulting in the intensification of social stigma against the disease. While its notification to city officials became mandatory, it was difficult to enforce due to the social stigma of infection and the economic consequences for the sufferer. In the 1950s, X-ray examination became a social ritual for Singaporeans, as it indicated good health and a necessary passage to stable employment for jobseekers. While the technology of mass screening became systemic, even outside hospitals and clinics, it created the social problem of the "X-rayed unemployable". While not infectious, these persons had traces of TB in their X-rays and were likely to be rejected by employers. It created a fear of radiography among the population that fed in turn into the existing stigmatization against tuberculosis (Arnold, 2003; Jie, 2020; Loh and Hsu, 2019, 2020).

The growing stigma attached to the sickness had a direct effect on public intervention and efficacy as it decreased the detection of TB in individuals and hampered the process of contact tracing. The problem of stigma-induced avoidance was especially high among the group of people most likely to have TB, as was underlined by the MOH in 1985. It seems that the stigma against the disease has been as resilient as the disease itself. Today, compared to many other countries, Singapore has not had great success in the elimination of TB. In spite of decades of public health education, the social stigma against TB remains present, deterring sufferers from seeking help and even affecting their livelihood after treatment. Singapore has passed legislation, mainly in the area of employment, to curtail stigmatization and its impact. Yet, much more needs to be done to educate the public on TB, precisely because it is widely regarded as an illness of the past. One lesson to take away from TB is that the root of its stigmatization is not pure ignorance of the disease but partial knowledge.

This, in turn, fuels people's fears and renders them immune to rational thinking. Ironically, hospitals can be a source of the stigma. Taking on the role of "moral entrepreneur", they can shape popular attitudes. For example, in the 1980s, medical personnel advised the separation of eating utensils at Tan Tock Seng Hospital and among family members in the home. This prompted some, notably older, Singaporeans to believe that tuberculosis could be spread through food, though this is not the case (Jie, 2020; Loh and Hsu, 2020; Yang, 2016).

Against this background, the COVID-19 crisis was treated very differently in terms of knowledge management. Instant-messaging groups enabled two-way discussion between frontline clinicians and MOH senior officials. The government has been careful to prevent misinformation by resorting to frequent and transparent public health communication. Uncertainties and gaps in knowledge were specifically acknowledged, leaving little space for false interpretations (Hsu and Tan, 2020).

Exaggerated fears of TB and other infectious diseases were to a large degree related to various official campaigns against public spitting in Singapore. These campaigns were successful, but they generated moral panic around spitting and highly stigmatized the spitter, setting them apart from the "civilized" community that Singapore was in the process of becoming. From the end of the nineteenth century onwards, moral panics have led to a "normative transformation" that altered ideas about the acceptability of spitting behaviour, thus redrawing society's moral boundaries. In fact, Singapore's anti-spitting movement has been an important factor for citizenship building in its socio-cultural history since colonial times. In a report published in 1907, the Municipal Commission pointed to "the habit of spitting so universal among the Chinese" as a cause of insanitation, tuberculosis, and pneumonia. Spitting in public places was prohibited under the so-called Anti-Spitting Ordinance. Nevertheless, spittoons remained common around Singapore. In his memoirs, Lee Kuan Yew recalled how difficult it was for the government to eliminate the practice after independence. In the 1950s, a nascent sense of civic consciousness arose among educated members of the public against spitting. At the end of that decade, health education efforts against spitting assumed greater national prominence and "anti-spitting exhortations contained the political vocabulary of self-determination and citizenship" (Loh and Hsu, 2020: 117). In 1956, the *Singapore Free Press* even drew a distinction between "civilized" people and "barbarians" who were spitting. In 1958, after the PAP won the City Council elections, the PAP mayor Ong Eng Guan launched a new campaign against spitting. In his own words, it was "an anti-social habit which does not conform to the self-respect of a people approaching self-government". While the new government was enforcing fines against offenders and condemning public spitting as anti-social behaviour, the Tuberculosis Control Unit (TBCU) partnered with the media to step up its anti-spitting education campaigns (Arnold, 2003; Jie, 2020; Loh and Hsu, 2020).

The 1980s saw a resurgence of moral panic surrounding spitting behaviours, notably with a strong public outcry in the media. An article in *New Nation* in 1985 described the act of spitting as "characteristic of an insensitive selfish individual", "nothing short of an act of barbarism", and "due to stupidity or lack of education" (Loh and Hsu, 2020: 118). The public outcry and the state campaign against spitting fed upon each other. Spitting was seen as spoiling Singapore's image as a modern and clean city. In 1984, the government began enforcing the anti-spitting laws by fining 128 people for spitting that first year and another 139 in 1985. Section 17(1)(g) of the Environmental Public Health Act, introduced in 1987, prohibits any person from spitting any substance or expelling mucus from the nose upon or onto any street or any public place (SSO, 2020). Moral panic around spitting created an institutional legacy of prohibition.

Interestingly, spitting continues to attract renewed attention from the public and the government with new outbreaks. For instance, with evidence showing that the virus that causes SARS was spread through droplets from the nose and mouth, the government mounted a new campaign in 2003 against spitting, took dozens of people accused of spitting in public into custody, and fined them $300 each (Arnold, 2003). Spitting also attracted renewed attention with COVID-19. In August 2020, a student was sentenced to nine months of probation because he had spat over a shopping mall railing in late February. The incident and the subsequent viral circulation of its video on social media happened just after the Disease Outbreak Response System Condition (DORSCON) was raised to Orange (Lam, 2020). This particular context and the way coronavirus spreads—through respiratory droplets, surface contact, and airborne transmission—were key factors in attracting media coverage and public attention towards spitting. *The Straits Times* even published an article in March 2020 reporting most of the spitting incidents that happened in the past weeks and related them to teenagers' behaviour (Chong, 2020b). Teenagers, Stanley Cohen's original folk devils (1972), became the new folk devils of the COVID-19 era in Singapore, at a time when the migrant clusters had not yet been discovered.

Moral panics and stigmatization can be observed with the outbreak of every new infectious disease, but to different degrees, according to the nature and infectiousness of the disease itself and the different socio-cultural attitudes present at a given time in society. Governmental action, cultural beliefs, and social attitudes play an important role in shaping the public perception of these infectious diseases. According to the Health Belief Model (HBM), the "perceived threat" of disease is composed of an individual's perceived susceptibility (or one's perception of how likely they will be infected) and perceived severity (or one's perception of how serious the disease is).

With a fatality rate of 14% in Singapore, SARS was a relatively high-mortality disease, yet the perceived severity of the disease during the epidemic in 2003 was low among the population. This seemed to be mainly due to the transparent and calm reporting of health authorities which provided the public with a continuous flow of information on the disease's evolution and the measures taken (Ibrahim, 2007; Ong and Yeoh, 2006). Posters, brochures, cartoons, advertisements, and a SARS dedicated TV channel provided information about the symptoms and transmission mechanism of the virus (James et al., 2006; Menon, 2006). While there were only 238 cases for a population of 4.1 million, the perceived susceptibility was high for SARS during the outbreak. People imagined that they could easily be infected by this "airborne virus that can spread through small droplets of saliva in a similar way to the cold and influenza" (World Health Organization, 2006). The SARS epidemic also brought about significant changes in the daily life of Singaporeans: They simply could not avoid being affected by it in some way or other. In its "risk communication" mode, the government seemed to be linking the SARS epidemic to global disasters and Singapore's national security, using war metaphors and martial language (such as "fighting a common enemy") to encourage social responsibility, as well as to strengthen identity and citizenship, drawing on the "siege mentality" discussed in Chapter 2. By emphasizing how every individual had a role to play in curbing the spread of the disease, the government made people feel more concerned about the disease (Ibrahim, 2007).

With AIDS, there was very high perceived severity among the population since the 1990s. In contrast to SARS, the perceived susceptibility among Singaporeans when it came to AIDS has been relatively low. The main reason behind this has been the strong tendency in Singapore to consider AIDS as peculiar to certain types of people, different from the "healthy" majority. According to the survey on attitudes towards AIDS in 1993, nine out of 10 of the respondents labelled PLWHA as "risk-takers" or "deviants" (Ong and Yeoh, 2006). In 2005, a junior health minister linked the "alarming AIDS epidemic" to gay parties and homosexual behaviours. By resorting to this kind of argument that is embedded in moral panics, he further stigmatized a category of people deemed deviant because of their alleged lifestyle. The overall negative image of AIDS as a disease associated with particular types of individuals and their presumed lifestyle weakened people's perception of susceptibility, as many considered their chances of being infected with HIV remote (Goh, 2008; Ong and Yeoh, 2006).

Another reason explaining the low perception of susceptibility towards HIV/AIDS is social taboo, the inhibition resulting from social custom or emotional aversion towards the disease and the way it is transmitted. According to the Ministry of Health, sexual intercourse remains the main mode of HIV transmission, accounting for 95% of all new cases, or 298 out of 313 in 2018 (Lee, 2019). Yet, Singaporean parents seldom discuss matters relating to sexuality with their children and many of Singapore's sex education programmes promote abstinence before marriage as the best protection against sexually transmitted diseases like HIV. Many Singaporeans might have questions that need answers, but sex remains taboo because of fears of being judged in a largely conservative society (Martin, 2018). Needle sharing, another way of contracting HIV, is also taboo as it is linked to the criminalized use of drugs.

Comparing SARS and AIDS reveals that an informed public tends to collaborate better and participate more effectively in containing the spread of the disease than a public in panic or shielded from the reality of the situation. In fact, high perceived susceptibility induces a general response and more prevention efforts from the people as they feel concerned about the disease. In order to enhance the population's perceived susceptibility to AIDS, health authorities should try to break the taboo on sexual intercourse and ensure the widespread diffusion of accurate and consistent information on HIV. They should also combat stigmatization of HIV-positive people, as it has discouraged public support for strong preventive efforts at the community and governmental level (Ong and Yeoh, 2006).

While SARS was a high-mortality and relatively less infectious disease, COVID-19 is a low-mortality and highly infectious disease. Yet, when it came to the perception of severity and susceptibility, and hence the perception of threat, it seemed COVID-19 was not very differently perceived as SARS. Raamkumar and colleagues (2020), studying public health behaviours through the lens of social media during COVID-19, extracted data from the Facebook pages of public health authorities, notably those of the MOH. Their study found that in the first 13 weeks of 2020, people talked more about susceptibility than severity (Raamkumar et al., 2020) as was the case with SARS.

This should not come as a surprise. First, SARS-CoV-2 and SARS-CoV are both coronaviruses (CoV) that present similar patterns of infectiousness. The World Health Organization described COVID-19 as spreading "primarily through droplets of saliva or discharge from the nose when an infected person coughs or sneezes" (World Health Organization, 2020). Not only do both viruses spread in a similar way, but they can also lead to acute pneumopathies. Second, the COVID-19 pandemic brought about significant changes in the daily life of Singaporeans, arguably even more significant than SARS. Third, the government resorted again to risk communication tied to national security, which eventually heightened popular concerns about the disease (Ibrahim, 2007). While these factors explain the high perceived susceptibility, the lower perceived severity can be explained by continuous and rather transparent flow of information on the disease's evolution and the measures taken by public health authorities. Once again, the government proceeded on the assumption that an informed and highly mobilized public could collaborate better and participate more effectively in containing the spread of the disease than a public shielded from the reality of the situation.

In the case of the COVID-19 pandemic, migrant workers in dormitories assumed the role of "folk devils" as they presented the doubly "deviant" characteristics of being by far the main group of people infected and of being foreigners. More about this will be discussed in Chapter 6.

SARS, A WAKE-UP CALL

In Singapore, there is a high level of socio-political trust, relative to many other countries (Abdullah and Kim, 2020; Woo, 2020; Ho, 2021). Much of this trust is based upon "performance legitimacy", which is built upon the state's continued ability to generate economic growth, ensure social stability, and deal with crises, including health crises (Woo, 2019). As far as public health is concerned at least, performance legitimacy comes regularly under threat, since a tropical and global city-state like Singapore, situated at the confluence of the movement of pathogens, is by nature vulnerable to outbreaks. The city-state and the government's survival both depend on their capacity to respond to public health emergencies and overcome them efficiently. While various outbreaks have tested Singapore's governance model, one in particular led to structural changes in health governance, producing an efficient disease response mechanism and a proactive approach towards the emergence of new outbreaks. SARS was that wake-up call for Singaporeans.

Tuberculosis (TB). After 1959, the PAP government elevated TB control to a national policy, building upon the foundational work done by the colonial regime. Its political commitment to combat the disease made available mass chest X-ray screening. The Housing and Development Board (HDB) and the Urban Redevelopment Authority (URA) also introduced public housing and urban renewal programmes to relocate people from overcrowded and unhygienic villages and slums to more sanitary residential areas and new towns (Teh, 1984). These efforts signalled to the public that the PAP government was determined to address the medico-economic issues affecting Singaporeans. Its anti-tuberculosis efforts helped the PAP to gain popular support (Loh and Hsu, 2020).

Singapore was successful in controlling TB, greatly reducing the number of cases over the decades. However, the current numbers seem to have stagnated compared to those of most developed countries worldwide, which have been declining. Between 2010 and 2019, between 1,978 and 2,791 new cases were detected each year in Singapore (Singstat, 2020). This can be explained by an ageing population and the increasing number of migrant workers from countries with high TB prevalence (Chee and Wang, 2012; Loh and Hsu, 2020). A few high-profile incidents of TB occurred in recent years such as the Parklane cybercafé cluster in 2012 and the Ang Mo Kio TB cluster in 2016 (Yang, 2016). In both situations, the MOH reacted swiftly to contain the outbreak, notably in providing onsite screening for the entire block with the use of a mobile X-ray bus, "a throw-back to the past" (Loh and Hsu, 2020). While these incidents put the disease under a spotlight temporarily, TB remains widely seen as an "illness of the past", a disease that occasionally challenges Singapore's health capacities and yet is mainly neglected by policymakers in comparison to other more "important" diseases. Yet, it is precisely this relative neglect of an infectious disease and the migrant population that it mainly affects that haunted Singapore in the case of COVID-19.

SARS. The outbreak of SARS in 2003 was a wake-up call for Singaporeans. The government's approach in dealing with COVID-19 drew heavily on its experience with SARS as well as further lessons it had learnt in dealing with the Chikungunya fever in 2008, H1N1 in 2009, and the Zika virus epidemic in 2016. Pointing to the role of SARS in enhancing Singapore's preparedness in the face of a sudden public health emergency, Prime Minister Lee Hsien Loong even declared in March 2020 that his government had been "preparing for this [COVID-19] since SARS, which was 17 years ago" (Lee, 2020).

The first case of SARS in Singapore was detected on 16 March 2003, followed by the issuance of a national travel warning to Singaporeans on 22 March. The same day, all SARS patients were moved to Tan Tock Seng Hospital (TTSH), whose medical staff were provided full medical protection. Schools were closed from 27 March to 6 April. From 31 March onwards, it was decided that all passengers returning from epidemic areas would be examined. Singaporeans with fever symptoms were sent to Tan Tock Seng Hospital. At the beginning of April, an epidemic prevention committee was set up to supervise the implementation of the response plan and coordinate the actions of ministries dealing with the disease (Lai and Tan, 2012; Tan, 2003; James et al., 2006). At the end of the SARS epidemic in August 2003, 238 people had been infected and 33 had died in Singapore, with a mortality rate of 13.9%, higher than China's 6.6% (Ooi and Phua, 2008).

The Singaporean government learned six crucial lessons from SARS that it translated pragmatically into key measures to strengthen its outbreak management capabilities.

First, the government enhanced hospital capacities and infrastructure dedicated to outbreak management. Before the SARS epidemic, there were only a few officials who paid attention to establishing institutional procedures to prevent hospitals and health workers from the threat of infection (Ooi and Phua, 2008). The previous infection prevention and control (IPC) measures mainly focused on infection during surgery and infection originating in hospitals. During SARS, the frontline medical workers were confronted with a shortage of complete personal protective equipment (PPE) (Chua, 2004, p. 21; Gopalakrishna et al., 2004). Due to lack of materials, experience, and preparation, SARS spread widely in Singapore's hospitals (Wong et al., 2020). In fact, about 74.8% of SARS cases were infected in hospitals, and 40.8% of the patients were medical staff (Ooi and Phua, 2008).

In the aftermath of the SARS epidemic, Singapore's hospitals formulated strict protocols and reconfigured facilities to prevent cross-infection among patients, visitors, and medical staff, which has now become standard protocols for daily practice. All newly recruited medical workers are now required to receive training in N95 mask installation and the proper use of PPE before starting work (Wong et al., 2020). Singapore established a six-month national stockpile of PPE, critical drugs, and vaccines. Furthermore, isolation facilities in public hospitals have been increased. The National Centre for Infectious Diseases (NCID), a "330-bed purpose-built infectious disease management facility with integrated clinical, laboratory and epidemiological functions", opened in September 2019. It replaced the former 39 isolation-bed Communicable Disease Centre (CDC) as the cornerstone of pandemic management in Singapore. There was expansion in the training of health care workers in outbreak response. As such, the number of infectious disease physicians rose from 11 in 2003 to 73 in 2020 (Lin et al., 2020).

Second, SARS prompted the advancement of research capabilities to study and take on infectious diseases. SARS was a turning point in the government's approach towards research on other infectious diseases such as AIDS, as it made the government realize that they cannot be simply overlooked. The government launched a joint research facility with the United States to conduct research on infectious diseases in the aftermath of SARS (Ong and Yeoh, 2006). Specialized institutions were set up, such as the NCID and the Duke-NUS Medical School. Researchers of infectious diseases in Singapore gained international respect. Some of these high-profile researchers, like Wang Linfa, director of the Duke-NUS Emerging Infectious Diseases Programme, were involved in the vaccine research for COVID-19. Singapore has also put more effort into adopting a multidisciplinary and collaborative approach to researching infectious diseases. The health capabilities include research areas such as genomics, molecular biology, data analytics, and bioinformatics (Sim, 2020). This, in turn, has created a "stronger ecosystem" to confront new outbreaks and viruses.

Third, SARS taught the government that clear leadership and direction were crucial for a comprehensive and coordinated response to outbreaks.

At the beginning of the SARS epidemic, the administration was overwhelmed and unable to cope with the unprecedented crisis. The MOH was hindered by its limited resources and could not get timely assistance and support from other departments (Ooi and Phua, 2008). A ministerial committee was therefore set up to provide guidance and decisions on strategies for containment of the outbreak. In fact, SARS led to the adoption of a more holistic whole-of-government (WOG) approach in crisis management. This WOG approach was crucial in subsequent outbreaks, including H1N1 and COVID-19, as it shortened the government's response time and facilitated health control implementation across various sectors (Lai and Tan, 2012; Lin et al., 2020).

During the COVID-19 pandemic, the government set up a multiministry taskforce only three days after Wuhan announced its lockdown. The taskforce, which followed the SARS model of the ministerial committee, included several Cabinet Ministers and was co-chaired by the then-Minister for Health Gan Kim Yong and the then-Minister for National Development Lawrence Wong.

Fourth, the SARS experience led Singapore to establish a proper disease response mechanism. The government set up the Disease Outbreak Response System Condition (DORSCON), which categorizes the domestic epidemic situation into four levels of incremental severity (green, yellow, orange, and red). Each level of threat corresponds to a set of public health measures and advice for the public. During the outbreak of H1N1 in 2009, the government, as a matter of precaution, raised the DORSCON alert level to orange on 28 April, even though there had been no local case in Singapore. The government then lowered the level to yellow 12 days later. Although this was criticized by a few clinicians as overly cautious, the preventive action of the government almost certainly had a part to play in the eventual reduction in the rate of community transmission (Singh et al., 2017; Lai, 2018).

In the case of COVID-19, when Singapore raised its orange alert in February 2020, people flocked to supermarkets to hoard essential supplies (Sim, 2020). This perhaps shows that while the legacy of SARS has been institutionalized by governmental agencies, the alert framework has had a stressful psychological impact on Singaporeans.

Fifth, the SARS episode made clear that public engagement and governmental attitude were essential components in the response to outbreaks. Throughout the pandemic, the Singapore government actively shared information with the public and kept raising public awareness on social responsibility (Menon and Goh, 2005). The SARS outbreak stressed the importance of political trust and communication for gaining public compliance with policies and regulations. These two factors explain political capacity in the context of Singapore and are interconnected, as "the public's willingness to accept the government's policy announcements [is] dependent on the presence of political trust and effective political communications further building up this trust and hence contributing to the government's political legitimacy" (Woo, 2020: 355). Overall, the government maintained a cautious attitude throughout the pandemic. On the same day that WHO announced there were no more SARS cases in Singapore, the government stated that "as long as there are SARS infected areas in the world, we cannot relax our vigilance" (WHO, 2006). Yan and colleagues (2006) argue that this cautious approach reflected the "survival" mindset of the government, which does not want to appear as letting its guard down. This careful attitude has been repeatedly displayed during the COVID-19 pandemic.

Sixth, rapid contact tracing followed by easily enforced quarantine was deemed critical in Singapore's successful containment of SARS. In the early stages, the MOH's epidemiological investigation work progressed slowly, resulting in the early failure to effectively cut off the chain of transmission. Most SARS cases were caused by local transmission. Only 8% of the cases were imported from affected countries (Ooi and Phua, 2008). Singapore's main strategy during this period was to conduct early detection of all cases and isolate all close contacts of symptomatic cases to prevent spread in the community. On 24 March 2003, Singapore revised its Infectious Diseases Act (IDA), the main legal basis for the prevention and control of infectious diseases. The revision enabled the government to implement compulsory quarantine for people infected with SARS and apply heavy penalties on those who violated the home isolation order (Menon, 2006). Yet, the MOH's resources were insufficient to handle the large number of Home Quarantine Orders (HQO). The law enforcement and surveillance work were eventually outsourced to a security agency called CISCO (Ooi et al., 2005). People ordered to stay at home had closed-circuit cameras installed in their houses to monitor their compliance with the quarantine order. Some viewed this as the actions of a "police state" in authoritarian Singapore (ABC, 2003). Others argued that prioritizing public interest over privacy concerns is consistent with Singapore's communitarian values (Menon, 2006).

To implement its contact tracing strategy, the MOH established a contact and tracking centre, which accommodated 200 officials at its peak, to quickly identify all SARS positive cases. This new system was however not able to cope completely with the rapid spread of the SARS virus. For example, from the SARS-related death of a worker in a wholesale market to the closure of that market, the authorities took a whole week to ensure that all those in contact with the worker had been quarantined (Chua, 2004).

Procedures detailing contact tracing processes were established in the aftermath of SARS. These procedures were eventually "encoded in the institutional fabrics of both the Ministry of Health and the NCID" (Woo, 2020: 350). The realization that contact tracing was key in responding to SARS paved the way for technological tools such as the TraceTogether app, a centrepiece in the response to COVID-19.

These six lessons from SARS were pragmatically and methodically institutionalized. Singaporeans came to realize more directly their vulnerability to regional and global epidemics. Since then, the authorities have enhanced its disease response mechanisms and adopted a proactive approach towards the emergence of new outbreaks. This has, in its COVID-19 response, proved to be effective, at least in the initial stages.

Conclusion

The next chapter discusses Singapore's efforts to tackle the COVID-19 pandemic. To understand the contradictions in these efforts, attention should be paid to at least three "public health" strands discussed in this chapter. First is the argument that Singapore's preparedness for COVID-19 was due in large part to the lessons well learnt from its experience with SARS. This had been a wake-up call that jolted the Singapore government into sharper awareness of the importance of building up healthcare and medical research capacity, leadership and public communication structures, and the ability to trace and isolate infections. Second is the argument that neoliberal globalization has, since the late 1980s, narrowed the focus of Singapore's public health to maximizing efficiency and optimizing the allocation of resources. This has made the healthcare system lean and, in that regard, less prepared for a crisis that would bring about a swell in demand for healthcare services. And third is the argument that Singapore's moralistic tendency to stigmatize groups of people reduces the seriousness and thoroughness with which disease management is extended throughout society, including its marginalized parts. The migrant worker dormitory outbreaks are a result of these contradictory strands.

REFERENCES

ABC. (2003). "Singapore Imposes Quarantine to Stop SARS Spreading", *ABC News*. https://www.abc.net.au/news/2003-03-25/singapore-imposes-quarantine-to-stop-sars-spreading/1823362.

Abdullah, Walid Jumblatt & Kim, Soojin. (2020). "Singapore's Responses to the COVID-19 Outbreak: A Critical Assessment", *The American Review of Public Administration*, 50(6–7), pp. 770–776. https://doi.org/10.1177/027507 4020942454.

Agence France-Presse (AFP). (2001). "Singapore-AIDS: Singapore a Third World Country for HIV Victims: Activists", *Aegis*. http://www.aegis.com/news/afp/2001/AF011193.html.

Arnold, Wayne. (2003). "In Singapore, 1970's Law Becomes Weapon Against SARS", *New York Times*. https://www.nytimes.com/2003/06/10/health/in-singapore-1970-s-law-becomes-weapon-against-sars.html.

Barr, Michael. (2020). "Singapore, the Limits of a Technocratic Approach to Healthcare", *Newnaratif*. https://newnaratif.com/research/singapore-the-limits-of-a-technocratic-approach-to-healthcare/share/cwguhz/97e3a2760 bbfebacf9d281c874939675/.

Chee, Cynthia Bin-En & Wang, Yee Tang. (2012). "TB Control in Singapore: Where Do We Go from Here", *Singapore Medical Journal*, 53(4), pp. 236–238. http://smj.org.sg/sites/default/files/5304/5304c1.pdf.

Ching, Sue Mae. (2020). "If I Get COVID-19, What Will I Need To Pay?", *Singsaver*. https://www.singsaver.com.sg/blog/what-will-i-need-to-pay-for-covid-19.

Chong, Clara. (2020a). "Drugs Used for HIV Treatment Now Subsidised by MOH", *The Strait Times*. https://www.straitstimes.com/singapore/drugs-used-for-hiv-treatment-now-subsidised-by-moh.

Chong, Clara (2020b). "3 Teenagers Arrested over Spitting Incident in Bugis Mall", *The Strait Times*. https://www.straitstimes.com/singapore/courts-crime/3-teenagers-arrested-over-spitting-incident-in-bugis-mall.

Chua, Mui Hoong. (2004). *A Defining Moment: How Singapore Beat SARS*. Singapore: Institute of Policy Studies and Ministry of Communications, Information and the Arts, Singapore.

Cohen, Stanley. (1972). *Folk Devils and Moral Panics: The Creation of the Mods and Rockers*. MacGibbon and Kee.

Department of Statistics Singapore (DOS). (2020). "Death and Life Expectancy—Latest Data". https://www.singstat.gov.sg/find-data/search-by-theme/population/death-and-life-expectancy/latest-data.

Foucault, Michel. (1980). *Power and Knowledge: Selected Interviews and Other Writings*. C. Gordon (Ed.). New York: Pantheon Books.

Goh, Debbie. (2008). "It's the Gays' Fault News and HIV as Weapons Against Homosexuality in Singapore", *Journal of Communication Inquiry*, 32(4), pp. 383–399.

Goh, Orlanda, Islam, Amina, Lim, John & Chow Wan-Cheng. (2020). "Towards Health Market Systems Changes for Migrant Workers Based on the COVID-19 Experience in Singapore", *BMJ Global Health 2020*. https://gh.bmj.com/content/5/9/e003054.

Gopalakrishna, Gowri, Choo, Philip, Leo, Yee Sin, Tay, Boon Keng, Lim, Yean Teng, Khan, Khan, Ali & Tan, Chorh Chuan (2004). "SARS Transmission and Hospital Containment", *Emerging Infectious Diseases*, 10(3), pp. 395–400.

Ho, Grace. (2021). "High Level of Confidence in Govt Here: Study", *The Straits Times*, 25 March. https://www.straitstimes.com/singapore/politics/high-level-of-confidence-in-govt-here-study.

Hsu, Li Yang & Tan, Min-Han. (2020). "What Singapore Can Teach the U.S. About Responding to Covid-19", *Stat*. https://www.statnews.com/2020/03/23/singapore-teach-united-states-about-covid-19-response/.

Iau, J. (2020). "Govt Clarifies Foreign Workers Under Covid-19 Quarantine Will Be Paid Salaries, Orders Correction of Facebook Post", *Strait Times*. https://www.straitstimes.com/singapore/courts-crime/govt-clarifies-foreign-workers-on-quarantine-will-be-paid-salaries-orders.

Ibrahim, Yasmin. (2007). "SARS and the Rhetoric of War", *Crossroads: An Interdisciplinary Journal of Southeast Asian Studies*, 18(2), pp. 90–119.

James, Shindo, Cutter, Jeffery, Ma, S. & Chew, Suok Kai. (2006). "Public Health Measures Implemented during the SARS Outbreak in Singapore, 2003", *Public Health*, 120(1), pp. 20–26.

Jie, Pan (2020). "How Tuberculosis Became a Chinese Disease", *Ricemedia*. https://www.ricemedia.co/current-affairs-features-epidemics-shaped-modern-singapore/

Lai, Allen Yu-Hung. (2018). "Agility Amid Uncertainties: Evidence from 2009 A/H1N1 Pandemics in Singapore and Taiwan", *Policy and Society*, 37(4), pp. 459–472.

Lai, Allen Yu-Hung, and Tan, Teck Boon. (2012). "Combating SARS and H1N1: Insights and Lessons from Singapore's Public Health Control Measures", *ASEAS—Austrian Journal of South-East Asian Studies*, 5(1), pp. 74–101.

Lam, Lydia. (2020). "Student Gets Probation for Spitting over Bugis Junction Mall Railing During COVID-19 Outbreak", *Channelnewsasia*. https://www.channelnewsasia.com/news/singapore/student-gets-probation-for-spitting-over-bugis-junction-mall-13053904.

Lee, Hsien Loong. (2020). "PM Lee Hsien Loong's Interview with CNN", *Prime Minister's Office Singapore*. http://www.pmo.gov.sg/Newsroom/PM-interview-with-CNN.

Lee, Joshua. (2019). "Number of Newly Reported HIV cases in S'pore Drops to Lowest Level in 14 Years", *Mothership*. https://mothership.sg/2019/07/hiv-statistics-singapore-lowest-2018/.

Lee, Vernon J., Chen, Mark I., Chan, Siew Pang, Wong, Chia Siong, Cutter, Jeffery, Goh, Kee Tai & Tambyah, Paul Ananth. (2007). "Influenza Pandemics in Singapore, a Tropical, Globally Connected City", *Emerging Infectious Diseases*, 13(7), pp. 1052–1057. https://doi.org/10.3201/eid1307.061313.

Lee, Yk. (1973). "Cholera in Early Singapore (Part I) (1819–1849)", *Singapore Medical Journal*, 14(1), pp. 1819–1849. http://smj.sma.org.sg/1401/1401smj11.pdf.

Lim, Meng-Kin. (1998). "Health Care Systems in Transition II Singapore, Part I: An Overview of the Health Care System in Singapore", *Journal of Public Health*, 20(1), pp. 16–22.

Lim, Meng-Kin. (2012). "Health Policy and Programming in Historical Perspective and Social, Political and Economic Context", in *Health Transitions and the Double Disease Burden in Asia and the Pacific*, edited by Milton J. Lewis, and Kerrie L. MacPherson. Taylor & Francis Group.

Lim, Janice. (2020) "After Years of Lobbying, Antiretroviral Drugs Used for HIV Treatment Now Subsidised by MOH", *Today*, 5 September. https://www.todayonline.com/singapore/after-years-lobbying-antiretroviral-drugs-used-hiv-treatment-now-subsidised-moh.

Lin, Ray Junhao, Lee, Tau Hong & Lye, David C. B (2020) "From SARS to COVID-19: The Singapore Journey", *The Medical journal of Australia*, 212(11), pp. 497–502.e1. https://doi.org/10.5694/mja2.50623.

Loh, Kah Seng & Hsu, Li Yang. (2019). "Tuberculosis in Singapore: Past and Future", *Annals of the Academy of Medicine*, Singapore 48(3), pp. 72–74.

Loh, Kah Seng & Hsu, Li Yang. (2020). *Tuberculosis—The Singapore Experience, 1867–2018: Disease, Society and the State*. New York: Routledge.

Martin, Mayo. (2018). "5 Things Singaporeans Want to Know About Sex—But Are Afraid to Ask", *CAN Lifestyle*, 18 May. https://cnalifestyle.channelnewsasia.com/wellness/singaporeans-sex-common-questions-spark-fest-asia-10235422.

Menon, Ku. (2006). "SARS Revisited: Managing Outbreaks with Communications", *Annals Academy of Medicine*, 35(5), pp. 361–367.

Menon, Ku & Goh, Kt. (2005). "Transparency and Trust: Risk Communications and the Singapore Experience in Managing SARS", *Journal of Communication Management*, 9(4), pp. 375–383.

Ministry of Education (MOE). (2011). "Governance Principles". www.moe.edu. sg/ne/AboutNE/GovPrin.html.

Ministry of Health (MOH). (2005). "Update on Singaporeans Infected with AIDS, Press Release", 1 December. http://www.moh.gov.sg.

Muzzati, Stephen L. (2005). "Bits of Falling Sky and Global Pandemics: Moral Panic and SARS", *Illness, Crisis & Loss*, 13(2), pp. 117–128.

Ong, Shir Nee & Yeoh, Brenda S.A. (2006). "HIV/AIDS in Singapore: State Policies, Social Norms and Civil Society Action", in *Population Dynamics and Infectious Diseases in Asia*, edited by Adrian C. Sleigh, et al. World Scientific Publishing Company.

Ooi, Giok Ling & Phua, Kai Hong. (2008). "SARS in Singapore—Challenges of a Global Health Threat to Local Institutions", *Natural Hazards*, 48(3).

Ooi, Peng Lim, Lim, Sonny & Chew, Suok Kai (2005) "Use of Quarantine in the Control of SARS in Singapore", *American Journal of Infection Control*, 33(5), pp. 252–257.

Quah, Elizabeth & Neo, Boon Siong. (2016). "Evolving the Governance of Public Healthcare Institutions—A Continuous Improvement Journey", in World Scientific. *Singapore health care system*.

Raamkumar, Aravind Sesagiri, Tan, Soon Guan & Wee, Hwee Lin. (2020). "Use 888 of Health Belief Model-Based Deep Learning Classifiers for COVID-19 Social Media Content to Examine Public Perceptions of Physical Distancing: Model Development and Case Study", *JMIR Public Health and Surveillance*, 6(3), e20493. https://doi.org/10.2196/20493.

Renia, Laurent & Ng, Lisa F.P. (2014). "Singapore's War on Infectious Diseases", *The Straits Times*, 28 November. https://www.straitstimes.com/opinion/singapores-war-on-infectious-diseases. Accessed: 5 November 2020.

Singapore Statutes Online (SSO). (2020) "Environmental Public Health Act". https://sso.agc.gov.sg/Act/EPHA1987?ProvIds=P1III-P4_17-

Singh, Shweta, Coker, Richard, Vrijhoef, Hubertus J.-M., Leo, Yee Sin, Chow, Angela, Lim, Poh Lian, Tan, Qinghui, Chen, Mark I-Cheng & Hildon, Zoe Jane-Lara. (2017). "Mapping Infectious Disease Hospital Surge Threats to Lessons Learnt in Singapore: A Systems Analysis and Development of a Framework to Inform How to DECIDE on Planning and Response Strategies", *BMC Health Services Research*, 17(1).

Singstat. (2020) "Population Death and Life Expectancy". *Singstat*. https://www.singstat.gov.sg/find-data/search-by-theme/population/death-and-life-expectancy/latest-data.

Sim, Dewey. (2020). "From Sars to Covid-19, What Lessons Has Singapore Learned?", *South China Morning Post*, 25 February. https://www.scmp.com/week-asia/health-environment/article/3052120/sars-covid-19-what-lessons-has-singapore-learned.

Tan, Bonny. (2020). "Cholera in 19th-Century Singapore", *Biblioasia*. https://biblioasia.nlb.gov.sg/vol-16/issue-2/jul-sep-2020/cholera#fn:21.

Tan, Chorh Chuan. (2003). "National Responses to SARS: Singapore", Presentation at WHO Global Conference on Severe Acute Respiratory Syndrome (SARS), 17–18 June 2003. http://www.who.int/csr/sars/confer ence/june_2003/materials/presentations/sarssingapore170603.pdf.

Teh, Cheang Wan. (1984). "Speech at the URA's 10th Anniversary Dinner on 30 March 1984". http://www.nas.gov.sg/archivesonline/data/pdfdoc/tcw19840330s.pdf.

Thomas, Joan Sara, Ong, Suan Ee, Chia, Kee Seng & Lee, Hin Peng. (2016). "A Brief History of Public Health in Singapore", in World Scientific. *Singapore Health Care System*.

Wong, Agnes Sau Kheng, Ooi, Chin Chin, Leow, Mabel Qi He, Kiew, Yen San, Yeo, Kenneth Chye Whatt, Tan, Soong Geck & Tay, Kiang Hiong. (2020). "Adapting Lessons From SARS for the COVID-19 Pandemic—Perspectives from Radiology Nursing in Singapore", *Journal of Radiology Nursing*, 39(3), pp. 164–167.

Woo, Jun Jie. (2019). *The Evolution of the Asian Developmental State: Hong Kong and Singapore*. Routledge.

Woo, Jun Jie. (2020). "Policy Capacity and Singapore's Response to the COVID-19 Pandemic", *Policy and Society*, 39(3), pp. 345–362. https://doi.org/10.1080/14494035.2020.1783789.

World Health Organization. (WHO). (2006). *SARS: How a Global Epidemic Was Stopped*. Manila: WHO Regional Office for the Western Pacific.

World Health Organization. (WHO). (2020). "Home/Health Topics/Coronavirus". https://www.who.int/health-topics/coronavirus#tab=tab_1.

World Bank. (2019). "Life Expectancy at Birth, Total (Years)—Singapore | Data". https://data.worldbank.org/indicator/SP.DYN.LE00.IN?locati ons=SG.

Yan, Jin, Pang, Augustine & Cameron, Glen T. (2006). "Strategic Communication in Crisis Governance: Analysis of the Singapore Management of the SARS Crisis", *The Copenhagen Journal of Asian Studies*, 23(1), pp. 81–104.

Yang, Hsu Li. (2016). "Remove TB Stigma to Better Fight the Disease", *The Straits Times*, 17 June. https://www.straitstimes.com/singapore/health/rem ove-tb-stigma-to-better-fight-the-disease.

CHAPTER 4

Tackling Covid-19, the Singapore Way

Johanna Dirlewanger-Lücke and Junhao Li

Abstract The Singapore government's strategy of managing the COVID-19 crisis in its first year was built upon its experience of handling the SARS crisis in 2003. The strategy showcased extensive capacities to test, trace, isolate, treat, and limit the importation of cases. Implementation was impressive at first, delivering results that were internationally admired. An emphasis on building social responsibility through transparent communication and the use of technology has also overall been successful. To keep the economy afloat and ready to thrive in post-pandemic times, the government allocated approximately $100 billion in a budget that was business- and employer-centric, consistent with neoliberal globalization. Where the government failed was in its handling of the disease outbreaks in migrant worker dormitories, which it seemed not to have anticipated even though there had been warnings from civil society

J. Dirlewanger-Lücke (✉)
Double Master Degree in Public Policy and European Affairs, National University of Singapore and Sciences Po (2021), Brussels, Belgium
e-mail: e0404064@u.nus.edu; johanna.dirlewangerlucke@sciencespo.fr

J. Li
Double Master Degree in Public Policy and European Affairs, National University of Singapore and Sciences Po (2021), Shenzhen, China
e-mail: e0404070@u.nus.edu; junhao.li@sciencespo.fr

K. P. Tan (ed.), *Singapore's First Year of COVID-19*,
https://doi.org/10.1007/978-981-19-0368-7_4

79

activists. Opportunistically, the PAP called for early parliamentary elections, arguing that a PAP government with a strong mandate was what successful management of this "crisis of a generation" required. Since Singaporeans are often thought to be risk-averse, there was an expectation of a landslide victory for the PAP with voters taking a "flight to safety" and supporting the only government they had ever known in this dominant-party system. Instead, the PAP lost significant vote share and 10 seats including two multi-member "group representation constituencies" were lost to the opposition. If these results reflected what voters thought of the government's performance in managing the COVID-19 crisis, they may well point more specifically to public dissatisfaction with immigration policy and the dormitories fiasco.

Keywords Pandemic crisis management · Testing · Isolation · Treatment · Public communication · Technology · General elections

Chapters 1 and 2 provided the political-ideological context of contemporary Singapore, which is simultaneously a nation-state and a global city. The legacy of small-state survivalism continues into the present and explains much of Singapore's proactive efforts to build capacity that can compensate for its constant nervousness about permanent vulnerability and fragile success. The turn to neoliberal globalization in the late 1980s explains the faith Singapore places in the market and the authoritarian role that the state plays in ensuring that the economy prevails over other considerations, which it views as highly dependent on a foundation of economic success. And that success, in a widely held belief, necessitates governance by a meritocratic, but increasingly elitist, government that is technocratic, pro-business, and pro-capital in the first instance and whose redistributive functions have been guarded and based on a cynical view of human nature. With the deepening of economic globalization and technological changes since the 1990s, and without a commensurate expansion of state welfare, income and wealth inequality has become a serious enough problem for the Singaporeans who have felt left behind to react more vigorously with frustration, anger, volatility, and an uncharacteristic level of criticality that is making the People's Action Party (PAP) government, in power since 1959, feel somewhat insecure. These are the starting points of a rise in authoritarian populism in Singapore, witnessed in the increasingly frequent examples of moral panic over the behaviour of elite figures in the establishment, of both elite and working-class foreigners, and of minority and marginalized communities in general.

Chapter 3 identified how these three strands—survivalist, neoliberal, and authoritarian populist—have shaped the public health choices and behaviours regarding tuberculosis, HIV/AIDS, and SARS in Singapore in recent decades.

In this chapter, we aim to describe Singapore's COVID-19 response measures and discuss how they have been shaped by these three strands in ways that create moral and policy blind spots. We conclude with a discussion of how the PAP government has responded to political and especially electoral pressures from Singaporeans whose experience of being left behind has been exacerbated by the pandemic.

The Singapore Success Story and Its Hidden Failures

"Singaporeans know what to expect, and how to react". These words were uttered by Singapore's Prime Minister Lee Hsien Loong in early February 2020, shortly before COVID-19 was declared a pandemic (Government of Singapore, 2020a). Early response by the government to contain the new coronavirus received international praise, making Singapore one of the countries that set the "gold standard" for COVID-19 response (Warrell, 2020). Yet, soon afterwards, Singapore was in the spotlight again, this time for a very different reason. The unexpected surge of cases and identification of several clusters in foreign worker dormitories at the end of March 2020 pushed the country into a "circuit breaker" that lasted for nearly eight weeks.

Where were the blind spots? And how could they have been missed by a government usually commended for its meticulous farsightedness?

More than a major health crisis, COVID-19 has caused immense disruption to economic and social systems nearly everywhere in the world. Interruptions in global value chains and a quasi-standstill of human mobility have magnified Singapore's vulnerability as a small island-nation. More than a decade earlier, Singapore's founding Prime Minister Lee Kuan Yew had already warned:

> Singapore cannot take its relevance for granted. Small countries perform no vital or irreplaceable functions in the international system. Singapore

has to continually reconstruct itself and keep its relevance to the world and to create political and economic space. (PMO, 2009)

Within a few decades after independence, the "little red dot on a map" became a global hub for trade, finance, and tourism. As discussed in Chapter 2, vast socio-political reforms and the embrace of neoliberal policies by a pragmatic top-down leadership transformed Singapore "from Third World to First". Today, The Singapore Story is a compilation of extraordinary economic achievements. The country's GDP per capita ranks among the highest in the world and solid growth has brought about major improvements in the quality of life of Singaporeans, including their health. COVID-19 has imperilled the narrative of continued success in The Singapore Story, raising uncertainties about what the next phase will look like.

Other than being a threat to public health and the economy, COVID-19 has exacerbated the symptoms of a deep-seated malaise in Singapore's socio-political system. The country's pursuit of neoliberal policies to attract multinationals and "foreign talent", while relying on cheap, low-skilled foreign workers to do the jobs that Singaporeans do not want to do, has resulted in growing social inequalities. COVID-19 shed light on one aspect of inequality through the government's bifurcated crisis response that separates migrant workers from the local "community".

It came to light that poor living conditions and lack of space in the migrant worker dormitories made safe distancing nearly impossible. The People's Action Party (PAP), Singapore ruling party since 1959, had ignored warnings by non-governmental organizations (NGOs). The dominant-party system has seen a paternalistic government, a weak civil society, scarce political opposition, and an obedient society engaged in limited deliberation.

At the same time, in the case of the Singapore "community", the strong PAP state could implement an efficient strategy to contain the virus through extensive testing, tracing, treatment, and isolation efforts, coupled with the comprehensive use of technology and government communication to encourage social responsibility.

FROM VULNERABILITY TO PREPAREDNESS

On 31 December 2019, the World Health Organization (WHO) China Country Office was notified about "cases of pneumonia of … unknown cause" in the Chinese city of Wuhan in the province of Hubei (WHO,

2020). Health workers were puzzled as patients showed a range of symptoms of varying degrees. Many of these patients had visited the city's bustling live animal market, where COVID-19 was presumed to have been zoonotically transmitted from animals to humans.

In 2003, 16 years earlier, the Severe Acute Respiratory Syndrome (SARS) virus was identified after the first cases of animal-to-human transmission had been reported in the southern Chinese province of Guangdong. That virus spread to 26 countries and killed 800 people. Most SARS infections were concentrated in East and Southeast Asia and within the healthcare environment. In only a year, the global outbreak came to an end through the "implementation of appropriate infection control practices" to end the chain of transmission (WHO, n.d.).

In early February 2020, a Ministry of Health (MOH) statement noted how the new coronavirus could "spread widely, resulting in a pandemic. This is the known unknown, and we have to assess what best to do" (MOH, 2020b). A week earlier, Singapore had reported its first imported case. The message was clear: like SARS, COVID-19 is a coronavirus transmitted by droplet infection and aerosols; and only by coordinated efforts to contain the disease as efferently as possible and prevent the importation of cases would a major health crisis in Singapore be avoided. The authoritarian political culture in Singapore enabled the government to take rapid measures, facing little opposition.

Singapore receives more than 19 million visitors annually, nearly four times its population (STB, 2020). Less than a month before a partial lockdown—dubbed a "circuit breaker"—was imposed, Prime Minister Lee had asserted: "We could not completely shut ourselves off the world" (Fan and Tan, 2020). In fact, having ties with many affected countries gave Singapore the advantage of international knowledge exchange where the virus was concerned, thus helping the Singapore government to make better-informed decisions (interview with Suan Ee Ong on 29 September 2020).

In a press conference over the coronavirus situation in Wuhan, then-Health Minister Gan Kim Yong was transparent about the inevitability "that we will see an imported case sooner or later" (Abu Baker, 2020). Singapore seemed prepared and confident. On 8 February 2020, Prime Minister Lee addressed Singaporeans:

We went through SARS 17 years ago, so we are much better prepared to deal with nCoV this time. Practically, we have stockpiled adequate supplies of masks and Personal Protective Equipment (PPE). We have expanded and upgraded our medical facilities, including the new National Centre for Infectious Diseases (NCID). We have more advanced research capabilities to study the virus. We have more well trained doctors and nurses to deal with this situation ... Most importantly, having overcome SARS once, we know that we can pull through this too. (Government of Singapore, 2020a)

Singapore's preparedness for the COVID-19 health crisis was to a large extent the legacy of SARS, as also discussed in the previous chapter. On the organizational front, the experience of SARS in Singapore led to adjustments to the country's crisis response capacities through the establishment of mechanisms to rapidly mobilize the government and the health sector. After SARS, medical personnel and health care workers received further training on how to respond to disease outbreaks. The success of a whole-of-government approach and the set-up of the Disease Outbreak Response System Condition (DORSCON) framework to coordinate ministerial and health authority efforts, as well as the creation of a 330-bed National Centre for Infectious Diseases (NCID) to isolate infectious cases have enabled Singapore to take swift action in the face of the COVID-19 crisis. In the words of Prime Minister Lee, Singapore has been "preparing for this" since SARS (Zakaria, 2020).

2 January to 6 February 2020: Early Response

Singapore reacted quickly to alerts by Chinese health authorities in early January 2020. Its geographical proximity to China and close "business travel, tourism and supply chain links" with China put Singapore at the forefront of the crisis (OECD, 2020). By 2 January, MOH issued a health advisory on precautionary measures regarding the situation in Wuhan, calling medical practitioners to closely monitor suspected cases of pneumonia. In order to limit the importation of cases, temperature screening machines at border checkpoints were installed. For example, at Changi Airport in Singapore, travellers from Wuhan were screened to detect fever. Two-week "stay home notices" (SHN) were issued for suspected cases that presented symptoms of pneumonia with a 14-day travel history to Wuhan. Singapore's early and proactive response, conditioned by its vulnerability mindset, took place even before China reported its first death, a 61-year-old man who died on 11 January. At this point in time, no instance of imported COVID-19 cases had been reported in Singapore.

On 13 January 2020, Thailand reported the first case outside of China. In the next few days, Japan and the Republic of Korea also reported cases imported from Wuhan. On January 2020, to strengthen its defence, Singapore extended the requirement for SHN to include travellers presenting symptoms and a 14-day travel history to China. On the same day, the United States reported their first case of COVID-19, prompting the Singapore authorities to reinforce vigilance by raising DORSCON from green to yellow.

In view of the degenerating situation in China and the increasing number of countries reporting cases, Singapore set up a Multi-Ministry Taskforce (MTF) on 22 January 2020 to step up its COVID-19 response. The MTF's job was to "plan and coordinate whole-of-Government efforts" in order to "mount a national response quickly and effectively" (MOH, 2020b). Co-chaired by then-Health Minister Gan and then-Minister for National Development Lawrence Wong and advised by Deputy Prime Minister and then-Minister for Finance Heng Swee Keat, the MTF represented 10 government ministries whose collective reach extended well beyond just public health. Through the MTF, Singapore was able to formulate targeted responses and coordinate important public communication. Notably, the MTF consisted mainly of the PAP's fourth-generation leaders—the so-called "4G leadership"—who were clearly being tested for their ability to manage a serious national crisis (Fisher, 2020).

One day later, on 23 January 2020, Singapore reported its first imported case. To put the events in Singapore into perspective, this happened the same day Chinese authorities announced an unprecedented measure to contain the disease in Wuhan by cutting the city off from the rest of the world. The images of the gigantic lockdown sent a strong message to the world that was "napping" (Kuguyo et al., 2020: 472). Shortly after, the WHO declared COVID-19 as a Public Health Emergency of International Concern (PHEIC). By 29 January, Singapore had detected 10 imported cases (MOH, 2020c). To strengthen efforts to test, trace, and isolate, authorities reinforced containment measures and deployed further testing capacities by opening screening centres at the NCID. Following the worsening situation in China, a further corner-stone in Singapore's strategy was established on 1 February 2020, as the country became one of the first to impose a travel ban for people coming from China.

Three days later, the first case of a locally transmitted infection was reported. In order to reinforce the detection of COVID-19 cases within society, testing capacities were made available at all public hospitals. In addition to those measures, Singapore extended temperature checks to the community level, with screenings being imposed at the entry of restaurants and shops, significantly reinforcing the country's capacity to detect cases (Kuguyo et al., 2020). Yet, in hindsight, the effectiveness of conducting large-scale temperature screenings is arguable, given the array of COVID-19 symptoms other than having a fever. There were also numerous cases of people with COVID-19 who showed no symptoms at all. Nevertheless, temperature checks were also reassuring, a visible sign that the government was taking action, regardless of its actual effectiveness.

In addition to those measures, each household received masks, which were mainly meant for those who had fallen sick. The Singapore Armed Forces (SAF) was also mobilized to assist the government with the distribution of masks and contract tracing, reinforcing the war analogies for "combatting" COVID-19 (Ng, 2020).

Did the Singapore public comply with the government's early response measures? Even in authoritarian political cultures, concerns over intrusion of privacy and other limits on freedoms cannot simply be ignored. The Singapore government therefore needed to ensure that the people were fully on board. For this, trust was a crucial component and communication was key (Joanne Yoong, personal interview on 29 September 2020). International surveys often show that the Singapore government enjoys a high level of trust among its citizens (Edelman Trust Barometer, 2020). Nevertheless, the government made considerable efforts to connect with its citizens during the crisis. For example, the Government Technology Agency (GovTech) used WhatsApp, a social media messaging platform used by nearly 4 million citizens, to provide daily updates on COVID-19. Through transparent and regular communication, citizens could feel more reassured (Basu, 2020). Research suggests that "balancing reporting on positively and negatively tested cases has been critical to keeping citizens calm through the epidemic" (Atmakuri, 2020). The government's online presence was also a way to fight the COVID-19 "infodemic". It provided guidance on its website on how to assess the truthfulness of COVID-19-related information, thus contributing to information hygiene.

There was also effort to ensure that public communication was comprehensible and assessable to all. For instance, the National University of Singapore's medical school produced "The COVID-19 Chronicles", a comic-book-style series of educational illustrations to inform the public about various important aspects of the virus in an entertaining and easy-to-understand way. However, this approach was not always successful. For example, the "Virus Vanguard", the government's comic series featuring a team of five COVID-19 superheroes, was criticized by the public for various reasons including the resort to offensive racial, gender, and class stereotype (Kamil, 2020). The comic was removed less than a day after it had been launched.

Overall, frequency and repetition of the government's call to be careful regarding misinformation was "key to increasing the salience and hence recall of the important facts, clarifications and behaviours [Singaporeans] should heed" (Soon, 2020).

7 February to 14 March 2020: Reinforcing Measures

As more cases were reported in the community, the government elevated DORSCON to orange on 7 February 2020, thereby heightening national vigilance. A week later the Public Health Preparedness Clinics (PHPCs) scheme was reactivated. Under this scheme, primary care clinic responses were consolidated into a single public health emergency framework to enhance crisis management capacities. On 17 February, COVID-19 testing capacities became available at all government outpatient clinics for patients presenting symptoms of mild pneumonia. With these measures, the government greatly reinforced its efforts to detect and isolate infected cases. Further action was taken to limit the importation of cases in reaction to the formation of clusters in South Korea and Northern Italy. The travel ban was extended on 4 March to these new "hotspots". As the virus had spread worldwide, the WHO declared COVID-19 a pandemic on 11 March.

In view of the dramatically worsening situation, Singapore had to find a way to ensure people continued to comply with the measures, without generating widespread panic. The government was especially aware of the problem of compliance fatigue. It drew heavily on behavioural insights. One of these is the notion that our brains are composed of automatic and

reflective systems. The first system allows us to make rapid, intuitive decisions. Often, we do them unconsciously. The second system enables us to
make reflective decision, by processing all information that is presented to
us. However, it takes time and is often effortful (Low, 2020). In the case
of COVID-19, people and governments were confronted with enormous
uncertainty and lack of time. Thus, the risk was that governments would
take quick, but poorly thought-through decisions. Also, group dynamics
influence our choice, making it harder to take the time to reflect on what
is truly the best response. This might explain the global "domino of lockdowns" that ensued. Instances of panic-buying around the world can also
be explained by this. Very soon after raising DORSCON to orange, Singapore experienced a wave of panic-buying, which prompted Prime Minister
Lee to deliver a televised speech transparently providing information and
urging Singaporeans not to rush to the supermarkets. To contain panic
within society, the public needed information and reassurance to make
more rational choices. Lee said:

> We have raised DORSCON to Orange before. You may not remember,
> but this was in 2009, for the H1N1 swine flu. So there is no need to
> panic. We are not locking down the city or confining everybody to stay
> at home. We have ample supplies, so there is no need to stock up with
> instant noodles, tinned food, or toilet paper, as some people did yesterday.
> (Government of Singapore, 2020b)

To fight behavioural fatigue, people needed to be constantly incentivized
to comply with the measures. They needed to easily understand and
remember the rules as well as how to use technology, which has been
designed to be as user-friendly as possible. This included smartphone apps
and QR codes to provide the latest information and updates, for reporting
daily temperature taking, for contact tracing, and for contactless payment.
Singapore's Smart Nation initiative, launched in 2014, was accelerated
during the COVID-19 pandemic, especially in its push for digitalization.

15 March to 6 April 2020: Managing the Panic

The COVID-19 trajectory took a turn when the disease shifted from an
external threat to a more clearly local problem. Measures to limit the
importation of the virus were inadequate for preventing the resurgence
of imported cases in the porous global city, as COVID-19 had become a

truly global problem. The government had to change strategy by reinforcing containment measures at home. Social distance measures were extended. The government banned large gatherings and enforced at least a one-metre separation between individuals in public spaces. At the same time, the travel ban was extended to European countries further away, such as Italy, France, Spain, and Germany. SHNs were issued to people coming from ASEAN countries, Japan, the UK, and Switzerland. On 23 March, all short-term visitors were eventually barred from entering or transiting in Singapore. Entertainment venues were closed. And social meetings were limited to 10 persons.

Amid the worsening situation in Singapore, a thicker climate of uncertainty and perhaps even of fear created the conditions that were ripe for moral panic and the tendency to scapegoat especially those who for whatever reasons did not or could not comply with government measures to control the pandemic locally. According to Stanley Cohen (1967: 9), moral panics are created when "a condition, episode, person or group of persons emerges to become defined as a threat to societal values and interests". This form of disproportionate collective panic may lead to "mass vilification" (Cohen, 1972: 11–12) of individuals and groups of people. In Singapore, amidst widespread fear and frustration, netizens in particular were prone to single out for public ridicule and shaming those who appeared to them to have flouted the COVID-19 rules. On Facebook, for example, was a very large group called SG Covidiots, where vigilante-style posting was quite commonly found especially in the earlier months of its existence. Some of these postings were explicitly xenophobic and racist. Alongside these social dynamics, an amendment was made to the Infectious Disease Act to introduce penalties for non-conformity with the rules. Those who broke social distancing or SHN rules risked jail terms of up to six months, fines of up to $10,000, or both.

The situation worsened greatly when several infectious clusters were identified in migrant worker dormitories. As Sulfikar Amir, a scholar of science, technology, and society, (2020) noted, the COVID-19 crisis "had uncovered a vulnerability Singaporean officials had not considered". This was a failure on the government's part to take fully into account the obvious high risk of contamination among dormitory residents. As will be discussed in Chapter 6, the poor living conditions of migrant workers have created the basis for rapid transmission. The crammed quarters did not enable residents to follow safe distancing measures adequately. The single-minded pursuit of neoliberal policies in Singapore had resulted in the exploitation and marginalization of migrant workers, even as they carried out the essential work of building and cleaning the wealthy global city. The failure to address the needs of migrant workers during this stage of the pandemic reflected a highly unequal society driven by capitalist principles.

CIRCUIT BREAKER AND THE TRANSITION TO A NEW NORMAL

At what must have seemed like the peak of the crisis, the government took the toughest action so far, which was to impose a two-month "circuit breaker", a partial lockdown which involved the closing of schools, workplaces, and public facilities to stem the transmission within society (Amir, 2020). After the end of the circuit breaker on 2 June 2020, Singapore cautiously embarked on its transition phase towards the new normal. The process was conceptually divided into three phases. Phase 1 began on 2 June 2020 and involved the safe re-opening of economic activities that presented no risk of transmission. Phase 2 began on 19 June 2020 and involved the resumption of most activities that could abide by strict safe distancing measures. Phase 3 began on 28 December 2020 and involved safe management measures and the heightened use of the TraceTogether app.

Singapore had launched this app on 20 March 2020, making it one of the first countries to introduce a tracing app. However, success was limited as only 1.4 million people downloaded it by August 2020 (Co, 2020). So, when it was announced that Phase 3 would be contingent upon 70% of the population downloading TraceTogether, fears over data privacy resurfaced as "data privacy laws in Singapore are heavily weighted in favour of businesses and government agencies" (Kaushik, 2020). The government repeatedly explained how the app worked, and it distributed tokens, initially targeted at the elderly, which could be used as an alternative to smartphones, reassuring Singaporeans that their private data would not be misused. Yet, in January 2021, government officials acknowledged that TraceTogether data can be used by the police for criminal investigations (Tham, 2021), which spurred debate in Parliament and among netizens. In February, an amendment to the COVID-19 (Temporary Measure) Bill was passed to clarify the circumstances under which data can be accessed by the police, providing a list of seven types of serious offences (Elangovan and Choo, 2021).

Singapore's COVID-19 strategy also involved providing financial support to businesses and households. Heng Swee Keat, Deputy Prime Minister and Minister for Finance at the time, presented the national budget—dubbed the "Unity Budget"—in Parliament on 18 February 2020, and subsequently announced additional packages to cushion economic shocks, address uncertainties, and prepare Singapore and Singaporeans for the future (Singapore Budget, 2020). The Unity Budget included a $4 billion "Stabilization and Support Package", which helped businesses to retain and support local workers. As the situation continued to worsen, a $48.4 billion "Resilience Budget" was announced on 26 March to provide support to households, further assist businesses to keep workers employed, and prepare the economy for its recovery. There were specific measures designed to support sectors hardest hit by COVID-19, such as aviation, tourism, food services, and the arts and culture (KPMG, 2020). One day before the circuit breaker, the government announced its "Solidarity Budget", a $5.1 billion stimulus package aimed at mitigating the impact of the lockdown. And then on 26 May, the government announced a $33 billion "Fortitude Budget" to support Singapore's transition to a new normal and prepare its economy and workforce for the future. The aim of this package was to stimulate the creation of jobs and strengthen the resilience of Singapore's economy by guiding businesses through future-proof transformation, such as digitalization.

In the first year of COVID-19, the government had already put aside close to $100 billion to cushion the economic impact of the pandemic, representing close to 20% of its GDP (EDB, 2020). The move was justified by the "exceptional circumstances" of the situation where "survival and existence are at stake" (Kurohi, 2020). But it did also send a strong message to Singaporeans of governmental support during this time of crisis and beyond (Suan Ee Ong, personal interview on 29 September 2020), which is a significant move for a neoliberal, welfare-adverse state (Tan, 2018).

A Covid-19 General Election: A Mandate for Action and Leadership Succession

Although it had until April 2021 to do so, the PAP government decided to call for early parliamentary elections on 10 July 2020, despite numerous proposals to postpone them until the coronavirus was stamped out. Senior Minister Teo Chee Hean explained:

Alternatively, a country can go for early elections, settle who will lead the country through this major crisis, give the new government a clear and fresh mandate, a full term ahead, legitimacy to take major decisions, tough decisions in the interest of Singaporeans. (Teo, 25 March 2020)

The government has described the COVID-19 pandemic and its economic fallout as "the crisis of a generation" (Lee, 7 June 2020). A snap election amid the COVID-19 pandemic could very likely be motivated by political opportunism. In conditions of uncertainty, the ruling party probably expected voters to take a "flight to safety", giving their votes to the only party with a track record in government, and a generally impressive one at that. In the words of Prime Minister Lee:

This General Election will be like no other that we have experienced. Not just because of the special arrangements to deal with COVID-19, but because of the gravity of the situation, and the issues at stake … These decisions will impact your lives and livelihoods, and shape Singapore for many years to come, far beyond the five-year term of the next government. (PMO, 2020)

GE2020 was also a test of the fourth generation or "4G" PAP leaders to see how they would manage a major crisis and what kind of support they could gain from the electorate. Although the election should not be seen as a referendum on the 4G leadership (Cheong and Zhuo, 2020), a "strong mandate" would endow the PAP with more confidence and capacity to proceed with the leadership transition.

The results of the elections were disappointing to the ruling party. Although it won 61.2% of the total votes, this was a drop from the 70% they had won in 2015. Furthermore, the Workers' Party, the leading opposition party, won 10 out of 93 elected seats in Parliament, the largest representation of parliamentary opposition since independence.

What would account for the relatively poor performance of the PAP, given the expectation of strong support for a government that has competently managed the COVID-19 crisis? One possible factor, among others, is the migrant worker dormitory situation. The outbreaks in these dormitories were more than a policy failure. They also exposed a fundamental weakness in the government: its inability to engage with alternative and opposition voices in a much more diverse and sophisticated society. NGOs had been warning the government about the living conditions in the migrant workers' dormitories, but they could not penetrate the PAP government's pragmatic and elitist mindset (George, 2017). As Cherian George and Donald Low (2020: 51) argue:

> The people who have been imploring the government to do more about the wretched living conditions of foreign workers have been vindicated; we should have been listening and paying more attention to them and their suggestions. They are our Li Wenliangs, and we are stronger as a society if we accept them as a legitimate and necessary part of our society, even if we disagree with them.

In response to the results, the PAP government explained—as it has always done—that it would engage in soul-searching, in an attempt perhaps to re-energize and reform (Tan, 2020). However, as Kenneth Paul Tan observes:

> The PAP has become decadent in a way that it has reached the zenith of its achievements and they find themselves utterly exhausted, ... the old theory of Singapore's success seems to have run its course ... GE 2020 ... certainly not the cause of political change in Singapore, but ... a reflection of a state of decline, the decline of a larger system and the PAP at the heart of this system. (Tan, 11 September 2020)

In Parliament, Prime Minister Lee admitted the government's mistakes in managing the health crisis in the foreign worker dormitories. Nonetheless, there was little to suggest that the PAP is going to change its policymaking style (George and Low, 2020).

While the survivalist orientation ensured that the PAP government stayed vigilant to pandemic threats confronting Singaporeans, and the neoliberal-globalization orientation motivated the government to take brave measures to keep the open economy going while allocating budgets out of its sizeable reserves to mitigate the pains associated with this, the same neoliberal outlook together with its authoritarian-populist reaction augmented the conditions of neglect towards the segregated community of working-class migrants. This blind spot, the site of Singapore's largest clusters of infection, will be the focus of the next two chapters.

References

Abu Baker, Jalelah (2020) "Singapore Forms Wuhan Virus Ministerial Task Force, Imported Case 'Inevitable': Gan Kim Yong." *Channel New Asia.* January 23. https://www.channelnewsasia.com/author/8700780.

Amir, Sulfikar (2020) "Hidden Vulnerability and Inequality: The Covid-19 Pandemic in Singapore." *Social Sciences Research Council.* October 22. https://items.ssrc.org/covid-19-and-the-social-sciences/disaster-studies/hidden-vulnerability-and-inequality-the-covid-19-pandemic-in-singapore/.

Atmakuri, Archana (2020) "Singapore's Fight Against the Coronavirus on Social Media." *InDepthNews.* May 9.

Basu, Medha (2020) "Exclusive: How Singapore Sends Daily Whatsapp Updates on Coronavirus." *GovInsider.* March 3. https://govinsider.asia/innovation/singapore-coronavirus-whatsapp-covid19-open-government-products-gov tech/.

Cheong, Danson and Tee Zhuo (2020) "Singapore GE: Elections Will Turn on Jobs, Covid-19 and Other Issues." *The Strait Times.* June 21. https://www.str aitstimes.com/politics/elections-will-turn-on-jobs-covid-19-and-other-issues.

Co, Cindy (2020) "Low Community Prevalence of COVID-19, 0.03% of People With Acute Respiratory Infection Test Positive: Gan Kim Yong." *Channel New Asia.* September 4. https://www.channelnewsasia.com/news/singapore/covid-19-singapore-low-community-prevalence-testing-13083194.

Cohen, Stanley (1967) "Mods, Rockers, and the Rest: Community Reactions to Juvenile Delinquency." *The Howard Journal of Criminal Justice,* 12.2: 121–130.

Cohen, Stanley (1972) *Folk Devils and Moral Panics: The Creation of the Mods and Rockers.* MacGibbon and Kee.

Economic Development Board (EDB) (2020) "Singapore Budget 2020: COVID-19 Relief Measures for Singaporeans and Businesses." June 23. https://www.edb.gov.sg/en/business-insights/insights/singapore-budget-2020--covid-19-relief-measures-for-singaporeans.html.

Edelman Trust Barometer (2020) "2020 Edelman Trust Barometer: Singapore." June 16. https://www.edelman.com/research/2020-trust-barometer-singapore.

Elangovan, Navene and Daryl Choo (2021) "Parliament Passes Bill Specifying Use of Trace Together, Safeentry Data by Police." *Todayonline.* February 2. https://www.todayonline.com/singapore/parliament-passes-bill-specifying-use-tracetogether-safeentry-data-police.

Fan, Jason and Tan Matino (2020) "PM Lee: S'pore 'Not Going to DORSCON Red' or Locking Down City Like The Chinese, South Koreans or Italians." *Mothership.* March 12. https://mothership.sg/2020/03/pm-lee-dor scon-red-no/.

Fisher, Dale (2020) "Why Singapore's Coronavirus Response Worked—And What We Can All Learn." *The Conversation*. March 18.

George, Cherian (2017) *Singapore, Incomplete: Reflections on a First World Nation's Arrested Political Development*. Woodsville News.

George, Cherian and Donald Low (2020) *PAP v. PAP: The Party's Struggle to Adapt to a Changing Singapore*. Singapore Academia.

Government of Singapore (2020a) "PM Lee: The COVID-19 Situation in Singapore." February 8. https://www.gov.sg/article/pm-lee-hsien-loong-on-the-covid-19-situation-in-singapore.

Government of Singapore (2020b) *PM Lee: The COVID-19 situation in Singapore*. March 12. https://www.gov.sg/article/pm-lee-hsien-loong-on-the-covid-19-situation-in-singapore-12-mar.

Kamil, Asyraf (2020) "Covid-19: Comic Superheroes Campaign Fails to Take Flight, Govt Says Sorry 'If We Offended Anyone." *Today Online*. April 20. https://www.todayonline.com/singapore/covid-19-comic-superheroes-campaign-fails-take-flight-govt-says-sorry-if-we-offended.

Kaushik, Preetam (2020) "Singapore's Approach to Protecting Citizens' Data Is Heavily Weighted in Favour Of Government And Businesses." *ASEAN Today*. February 20. https://www.aseantoday.com/2020/02/singapores-approach-to-protecting-citizens-data-is-heavily-weighted-in-favour-of-government-and-businesses/.

KPMG (2020) "Singapore. Government and Institution Measures in Response to COVID-19." September 9. https://home.kpmg/xx/en/home/insights/2020/04/singapore-government-and-institution-measures-in-response-to-covid.html.

Kuguyo, Oppah, Andre P. Kengne, and Collet Dandara (2020) "Singapore COVID-19 Pandemic Response as a Successful Model Framework for Low-Resource Health Care Settings in Africa?" *OMICS: A Journal of Integrative Biology*, 24.8: 470–478.

Kurohi, Rei (2020) "Coronavirus: S'pore's Survival and Existence at Stake, Draw on Reserves Needed to Take Care of People, Says President." *The Straits Times*. May 22. https://www.straitstimes.com/singapore/coronavirus-spores-survival-and-existence-at-stake-draw-on-reserves-needed-to-take-care-of.

Lee, Hsien Loong (2021) "Overcoming the Crisis of a Generation." June 7. https://www.gov.sg/article/pm-lee-hsien-loong-overcoming-the-crisis-of-a-generation.

Lin, Ray Junhao, Lee, Tau Hong and Lye, David CB (2020). "From SARS to COVID-19: The Singapore Journey." *Medical Journal of Australia*, 212.11: 497–502.

Low, Donald (2020) *Behavioural Economics and Policy Design. Examples from Singapore*. World Scientific Publishing.

Ministry of Health (MOH) (2020a) "Multi-Ministry Taskforce on Wuhan Coronavirus. Terms of Reference (TORs) and Composition." https://www. moh.gov.sg/docs/librariesprovider5/default-document-library/multi-min istry-taskforce-on-wuhan-coronavirus-and-tor---final.pdf.

Ministry of Health (MOH) (2020b) "Ministerial Statement on Whole-Of-Government Response to the 2019 Novel Coronavirus (2019-Ncov)." February 3. https://www.moh.gov.sg/news-highlights/details/ministerial-statement-on-whole-of-government-response-to-the-2019-novel-coronavirus-(2019-ncov).

Ministry of Health (MOH) (2020c) "Three More Confirmed Imported Cases of Wuhan Coronavirus Infection in Singapore." January 29. https://www. moh.gov.sg/news-highlights/details/three-more-confirmed-imported-cases-of-wuhan-coronavirus-infection-in-singapore.

Ng, Vivian (2020) "How Singapore's Military Is Fighting COVID-19." *The Diplomat.* March 24. https://thediplomat.com/2020/03/how-singapores-military-is-fighting-covid-19/.

Organisation for Economic Co-operation and Development (OECD) (2020) "COVID-19 crisis response in ASEAN Member States." May 4. https:// www.oecd.org/coronavirus/policy-responses/covid-19-crisis-response-in-asean-member-states-02f828a2/.

Prime Minister's Office (2009) "Speech by Mr Lee Kuan Yew, Minister Mentor, at the S. Rajaratnam Lecture." 09 April 2009, 5:30 pm at Shangri-La Hotel. https://www.pmo.gov.sg/Newsroom/speech-mr-lee-kuan-yew-minister-mentor-s-rajaratnam-lecture-09-april-2009-530-pm-shangri.

Prime Minister's Office (2020) "Speech on General Election 2020 by PM Lee Hsien Loong." June 23. https://www.pmo.gov.sg/Newsroom/Speech-on-GE2020-by-PM-Lee-Hsien-Loong.

Singapore Budget. (2020) "Budget 2020: Budget Measures." https://www.sin gaporebudget.gov.sg/budget_2020/budget-measures.

Singapore Tourism Board (STB) (2020) *Tourism Sector Performance. Q4 2019 Report.*

Soon, Carol. (2020) "Fighting an Information Avalanche During Covid-19 Outbreak." *Todayonline.* March 17. https://www.todayonline.com/commen tary/fighting-information-avalanche-covid-19-outbreak-fake-news-WhatsApp.

Tan, Kenneth Paul (2018) *Singapore: Identity, Brand, Power.* Cambridge University Press.

Tan, Kenneth Paul (2020) "Singapore's GE2020: The Real Watershed Election? [Webinar]." The Malaysia and Singapore Society of Australia (MASSA). September 11. https://www.facebook.com/watch/live/?v=261691108181 324&ref=watch_permalink.

Teo, Chee Hean. (2020) "Reply in Parliament on the Impact of COVID-19 on the General Election." March 25. https://www.pmo.gov.sg/Newsroom/ SM-Teo-Chee-Hean-reply-in-Parliament-on-the-impact-of-COVID-19-on-the-GE.

Tham, Yuen-C (2021) "Police Can Use Trace Together Data for Criminal Investigations." *The Straits Times*. January 5. https://www.straitstimes.com/singap ore/politics/police-can-use-tracetogether-data-for-criminal-investigations-0.

Warrell, Margie (2020) "COVID-19 Leadership Lessons From Singapore: Be Ready, Be Bold, Be Decisive." *Forbes*. March 30. https://www.forbes. com/sites/margiewarrell/2020/03/30/singapore-sets-gold-standard-aga inst-covid-19-be-ready-be-decisive-be-bold/?sh=59a8576d7a22.

World Health Organization (WHO) (2020) "Pneumonia of Unknown Cause— China." January 5. https://www.who.int/csr/don/05-january-2020-pne umonia-of-unkown-cause-china/en/.

World Health Organization (WHO) (n.d.) *Severe Acute Respiratory Syndrome (SARS)*.

Zakaria, Fareed (2020) "On GPS: What the U.S. can Learn from Singapore on Covid." *CNN International.* March 29. https://edition.cnn.com/vid eos/tv/2020/03/29/exp-gps-0329-loong-on-what-us-can-learn-from-sin gapore.cnn.

CHAPTER 5

The Contradictions and Challenges of Singapore's Immigration Policy

Davide Brugola and Michael Flood

Abstract Immigration policy in cosmopolitan Singapore focuses on two separate flows: one of foreign talent and the other of migrant workers. The ruling People's Action Party (PAP) government's pragmatic, which has come to really mean dogmatically neoliberal, approach to immigration policy has been shaped by the Great Recession of 2007–2009, relatively disappointing results in the 2011 general elections, and popular reactions to a 2013 population white paper that pointed to a more crowded future with greater numbers of foreigners in the global city. In response to popular pressure against excessive inflow of foreigners, the government tends to express empathy in public communication and make marginal revisions to the policy, while adamantly pursuing a neoliberal agenda that

D. Brugola (✉)
Double Master Degree in Public Policy and European Affairs, National University of Singapore and Sciences Po (2021), Carbonate, Italy
e-mail: e0404068@u.nus.edu; davide.brugola@sciencespo.fr

M. Flood
Double Master Degree in Public Policy and European Affairs, National University of Singapore and Sciences Po (2021), Paris, France
e-mail: e0404071@u.nus.edu; michael.flood@sciencespo.fr

99

keeps Singapore profitably reliant on foreign labour. The "Little India riot", which exploded in a crowded district where South Asian migrant workers congregated on their days off, pointed to the untenability of this policy approach. And yet, not much has changed subsequently, leading to the vivid exposure of the system's vulnerability when it was confronted with an unexpected global public health crisis in 2020.

Keywords Immigration policy · Foreign talent · Migrant workers · Great Recession 2007–2009 · General elections · Population White Paper · Little India riot

Immigration to the island-state of Singapore is one important piece of a larger mosaic of economic policymaking aimed at maintaining the city's viability, relevance, and attractiveness on the global stage. Singapore is a cosmopolitan destination with all the bells and whistles of the most advanced cities in the world. An increasing inflow of foreign talent in the past two decades has transformed Singapore into a prized destination for high salaries and all the lifestyle options that such salaries can afford. Foreign academics and international students have helped to create the semblance of a "global knowledge enterprise" (Sidhu et al., 2011). These and other trends can helpfully be understood through the lens of neoliberal globalization.

Even before Singapore had become independent, its first Prime Minister Lee Kuan Yew was already able to articulate a materialistic vision of politics that belittled the ideals of liberal democracy and its political institutions:

> The mass of the people are not concerned with legal and constitutional forms and niceties. They are not interested in the theory of the separation of powers and the purpose and function of a politically neutral public service ... If the future is not better, either because of the stupidities of elected ministers or the inadequacies of the civil servants, then at the end of the five-year term the people are hardly likely to believe either in the political party that they have elected or the political system that they have inherited. (Lee, 1959)

After independence in 1965, Singapore moved towards becoming an export-oriented economy, reaching full employment by the 1970s, before eventually aspiring towards a "knowledge-based economy" (KBE) in the 1980s and 1990s (Low, 2002). The open-door policy to skilled, semi-skilled, and unskilled labour was formalized in the 1970s when Singapore experienced major shortages in manufacturing and construction (Dobbs and Loh, 2019). Initially, many of these workers came from Malaysia, including an increasing number of women who by 1978 had taken over males in the manufacturing industry largely due to increased production of garments and textiles.

By the end of the 1990s, the only metric on which Singapore fell short of its developed-economy comparators, largely in the West, was educational achievement (Low, 2002: 96). To address that, the "global schoolhouse" initiative was launched in 2002 as the last piece needed to complete the KBE puzzle, and to cement Singapore as a highly skilled, highly sought-after destination for the world's brightest. Partnerships with universities like MIT were established and the National University of Singapore was remodelled into an elite, global university (Sidhu et al., 2010). An estimated 60% of academics in Singapore's universities are foreign-born (Paul and Long, 2016).

Singapore continued to attract highly skilled foreign talent. The percentage of skilled workers in 1988 was around 19%, increasing to 34% just 10 years later. As the turn of the millennium drew nearer, policies were implemented to reach a target of 65% in the following 10 or 15 years (Ministry of Manpower, 1999). Between the period of 2004 and 2009, the Permanent Resident (PR) population grew at an annualized rate of 8.4% versus just 0.9% for Singapore citizens (Migration Policy Institute, 2012). In spite of some unfavourable public sentiment, the government has not really curbed plans to bring in more foreign talent. On the contrary, it has recently articulated the need to attract even more foreign professionals, managers, executives, and technicians (PMETs) as part of its economic development agenda, Industry 4.0 (The ASEAN Post, 2020).

The issue goes beyond the need to populate the workplace. Strikingly low fertility rates among residents, especially among ethnically Chinese Singaporeans, have created a need to adequately populate the nation. The rates began plummeting in the late 1970s and hit a low in 1976 of 1.15 births per woman before dropping further to as low as 1.05 among local Chinese women by 2010 (Yeoh and Lin, 2013). Immigration policy has in many ways been a response to declining birth rates as much as it has been about the city-state's transformation into a hub of enterprise and knowledge.

Currently, after the outbreak of COVID-19, the foreign workforce comprises over 34% of the total working population of 3.6 million, and roughly a quarter of the total population of 5.69 million, even after a large outflow of about 200,000 migrant workers following the pandemic (Department of Statistics, 2020). This foreign workforce actually consists of foreign talent, on the one hand, and low- and semi-skilled migrant workers, on the other. Singaporean economist Linda Low (2002) describes the growth of these migrant workers in the 1980s, when Singapore underwent an aggressive industrialization phase propping up its construction and manufacturing sectors through the attraction of unskilled, foreign workers in largely "dirty, demeaning, and dangerous jobs". The migrant workforce consists of Work Permit holders in construction, manufacturing, marine shipyard, service and process sectors, as well as foreign domestic workers (FDWs) who are almost entirely women living and working in-house. It is estimated one in five households in Singapore employs a live-in FDW (MOM, 2020).

Table 5.1 shows how Singapore's foreign workers are classified under the Employment Act, enforced by the Ministry of Manpower (MOM). Work Permit holders, by far the largest portion of foreigners working in Singapore, are entitled to little more than the right to work for a registered employer. Moving up the scale, S Pass holders have some technical skills and a salary of at least $2,500. Their numbers have sharply increased in the last five years with an additional 30,000 holders registered with MOM. Employment Pass holders have also surged, although it is not reported how these numbers are divided along EP and PEP lines, the latter referring to the "C-Suite" executives taking up some of the nation's most coveted and lucrative positions.

In 2013, the government released its Population White Paper that stated 6.9 million as a population planning parameter for 2030. This would require 100,000 immigrants per year. More liberal immigration policies since the mid-2000s have radically altered Singapore's social fabric. These rising numbers have triggered local pressure to moderate this reliance on foreigners and prioritize Singaporeans instead (Bloomberg, 2020). Prime Minister Lee Hsien Loong has responded by urging equanimity amid protectionist sentiments catching fire across developed economies (Reuters, 2020). In November 2020, the government announced a new "Tech.Pass" programme to draw in the top talent in the information technology sector, aiming to attract an initial cohort

Table 5.1 Classification of foreign employment in Singapore

	Work Permit	S Pass	Employment Pass	Personalized Employment Pass
Income Requirement (monthly)	N/A	Min. $2,500	Min. $4,500 $5,000 for financial services (2 × the min. for candidates in their 40s and older)	Min. $12,000 for current EP holders Min. $18,000 for overseas professionals
Family Allowance	N/A	Passes available for spouse, children when income exceeds $6,000	Passes available for spouse (must be legally married, otherwise a Long-Term Visit Pass (LTVP) is required, normally only issued to Singaporean Citizens or Permanent Residents) and children when income exceeds $6,000 LTVP for parents when income exceeds $12,000	Passes available for spouse and children when income exceeds $6,000 Long-Term Visit Pass (LTVP) for parents when income exceeds $12,000
Restrictions and Barriers to Entry	Non-transferrable Must not operate a business or earn supplemental income No marrying a Singaporean or PR without MOM approval No pregnancy unless married to Singaporean or PR with approval	Must hold a degree or diploma Relevant work experience	Acceptable qualifications, usually defined as University Degree Must meet PMET job specifications	Cannot go unemployed for 6+ months at any time while in Singapore No freelancers, journalists, editors, or producers Cannot start a business (requires EntrePass)
Labour Profile	Construction, Foreign Domestic Work, Manufacturing, etc	Diploma Holders	Professionals, Managers, Executives, and Technicians (PMETs)	High-Income Executives ("C-suite")

(continued)

Table 5.1 (continued)

	Work Permit	S Pass	Employment Pass	Personalized Employment Pass
Number of Holders (December 2019)	2014: 991,300 2019: 999,000 (0.8% growth)	2014: 170,100 2019: 200,000 (15% growth)	2014: 178,900 2019: 193,700 (8.3% growth)	Included in Employment Pass statistics

Source Ministry of Manpower (2020) Foreign Workforce Numbers. Available at https://www.mom.gov.sg/documents-and-publications/foreign-workforce-numbers

of up to 500 tech executives and entrepreneurs who must meet salary requirements of at least $20,000 in order to obtain the two-year visa (Bloomberg, 2020).

Foreign Talent

Lured by Singapore's cosmopolitan attractiveness and high salaries, foreign talents have come in large numbers (Teo, 2019). HSBC/YouGov's Expat Explorer survey has ranked Singapore as the best destination for expatriating families for many years running, falling second place to Switzerland in the most recent issue. The 2020 guide highlighted what expats consider to be the most promising features of Singapore as a work-life destination: political and economic stability, quality of life and education, and good outcomes for career progression. Upon arrival, respondents reported an increased sense of safety and increased well-being for their children, but they also reported less satisfaction with cultural values, notably the work-life balance and ease of making acquaintances. There remains, however, a utopian conception of Singapore that is all but confirmed for the highly talented, highly mobile families who choose to call the city-state home.

The practice of attracting high-skilled talent to prop up the national economy is not unique to Singapore. In an extensive review of available data, Kerr and colleagues (2016) explain the pull factors for global talent flows in recent times, noting that policymakers in developed countries have recognized the need for increased human capital to fuel their growth trajectories. Singapore, the authors observe, is small and nimble enough to adopt a strategy of "immigration engineering", fluctuating inflows based on market demand and public sentiment (Kerr et al., 2016: 15).

Indeed, attracting high-skill talent is part of calculated reforms that go back decades. Terri-Anne Teo (2019), a Singaporean political scientist and commentator on civic multiculturalism in Singapore, describes the form of cosmopolitanism co-opted by Singapore—one that is more about a globally lavish lifestyle and less about supranational democratic values— as an effort to attract and retain foreign talent. Foreign talent is seen as a form of symbolic capital contributing to the state's economic engine, which is evidenced in the state's multi-tiered foreign talent policy. In a rhetorical defence of this, the government issued a statement in July 2020 explaining why—even with an increasingly educated Singaporean work-force—foreign talent must be retained (Government of Singapore, 2020). The jobs they help to create, the government argues, are needed for Singaporeans to achieve their "career aspirations" and they can "upgrade their skills to eventually take on these higher paying jobs".

Yet, taken as part of a larger mosaic, foreign talents do not readily fit into Singapore society. Yang (2018) takes a Lacanian psychoanalytic view in arguing that ordinary Singaporeans have a rather less positive idea about foreign talent. Foreigners doing low and medium pay work (mainly, Work Permit and S Pass holders) and foreign students on government scholarships underperforming relative to their Singaporean counterparts are all the proof needed to suggest that much of the "imported talent" is "downright bogus" (Yang, 2018: 1024). What is at issue, Yang argues, is the idea that while foreign talent is to represent the ideals and symbols—the "knowledge"—that Singapore and Singaporeans lack, their arrival is met with disappointment, leaving the desires of Singaporeans unmet and empty. Instead, there is resentment for their new compatriots (Yang, 2018: 1025–1027).

There are, in fact, policies in place to address the issue that Singaporeans might unfairly lose out to their foreign counterparts as far as job opportunities are concerned. Firms must abide by the Fair Consideration Framework (FCF), which monitors hiring activities along ethno-demographic lines and ensures that a proper merit-based process is pursued. As of October 2020, all employment agencies operating in Singapore are required to comply with the Tripartite Guidelines on Fair Employment Practices (TGFEP). Working around the rules—including the requirement to make "reasonable efforts to attract Singaporeans for vacancies that they are trying to fill"—could result in agencies having their licence suspended or revoked. While these measures are a real response to increased public pressure to fill vacancies with Singaporean nationals, it is unclear how effective they are in practice and the extent to which protocols are taken seriously and actually enforced.

Migrant Workers

Low- and semi-skilled migrant workers make up the second flow of immigrant workers in Singapore. Consisting of about a million workers or roughly one in three in the Singapore workforce, migrant workers mostly come from Bangladesh, Malaysia, China, and India. They are offered two-year renewable Work Permits, sponsored by local companies that agree to hire them, and work mainly in five sectors: construction, manufacturing, marine shipyard, processing, and service (Ministry of Manpower, 2018).

While there is no minimum monthly salary, employers must declare to MOM the salaries they will pay. They are responsible for ensuring their workers have access to housing and some basic medical insurance. And, with the exception of Malaysian workers, employers must purchase a $5,000 security bond, which functions as a deposit guaranteeing that the Work Permit will not be broken by the employer or the worker.

Migrant workers' responsibilities include not seeking any employment except that which is stipulated by the permit, not opening a business, not marrying a Singaporean citizen, and not getting pregnant. If the work permit is terminated, the worker must be repatriated and bear the costs of it. According to a MOM survey of 3,045 respondents (2,523 Work Permit holders and 522 S Pass holders) conducted in 2018, more than three-quarters of Work Permit holders planned to continue working in Singapore after their current contracts expired. A further 13% planned to return home before coming back to Singapore again for work, a rate that has more than doubled since 2014. The same study found that 84 per cent of Work Permit holders and 91% of S Pass holders would recommend living and working in Singapore to a friend. The top five reasons for recommendation are listed in Table 5.2

Table 5.2 Migrant workers reasons for recommending Singapore as a place to live/work

Reasons most commonly cited	WP Holders (%)		S Pass Holders (%)	
	2014	2018	2014	2018
Top five reasons for recommending Singapore as a place to work (multiple options allowed)				
Good pay	71.7	67.0	71.8	74.7
Safe and secure country	35.4	62.6	39.1	74.3
Good living conditions	34.2	55.7	51.0	75.4
Good working conditions	44.3	48.1	52.8	66.9
Good prospects	19.0	29.3	16.6	31.4

Source Ministry of Manpower Foreign Worker Experience Survey, 2018

Except for Work Permit holders' perceptions about pay, on all other aspects, there was improvement from 2014 to 2018. Singapore is still viewed by migrant workers as a "land of opportunity", as seen in a headline in *The Straits Times* (October 2020). In the article, Rahim, a worker who has been employed under the Work Permit programme since 1999, describes the wealth he has amassed since his arrival and how the remittances sent to his wife and daughter are enough to support them, with money remaining for investments and upskilling.

The "land of opportunity" narrative is often referred to whenever migrant workers' conditions of living and working are criticized in Singapore. National newspapers often post stories about how migrant workers are grateful to Singaporeans for their care and hospitality. "Moved by the care migrant worker pens grateful Facebook note" reads a piece in *The Strait Times* from May 2020. The article closes with the worker who had contracted COVID-19 asserting that when he recovered, he hoped to "work hard and contribute back to Singapore". Many Singaporeans take these expressions of gratitude literally, without critically considering the precarious conditions within which migrant workers are forced to behave in acceptable ways.

Foreign domestic workers (FDWs) are perhaps caught in even more precarious conditions. Their work falls outside the reach of the Employment Act as it has been considered too impractical for MOM to regulate work of a domestic nature, requiring monitoring of hours worked, what is expected on their days off, and so on (Poh, 2016). Even more restricting is the incapacity to quit or terminate a contract at the domestic workers' discretion. The employer must consent to their release either to repatriate or transfer to another employer (Poh, 2016: 6). Moreover, employers can cancel FDW contracts at a moment's notice. Evidence collected by Singaporean civil society organization, Humanitarian Organization for Migration Economics or HOME (2017), suggests that live-in workers are generally confined to living quarters of a few square metres, if given a separate room, and can be made to sleep in the kitchen quarters on a mat or thin mattress if space is tight. Moreover, many report having surveillance cameras installed in their quarters and limited or no access to a private space to store or lock belongings.

While busy building its global brand as a talent hub in Southeast Asia, Singapore has adopted a strategy to ensure a sufficient supply of manual labour to do the kind of jobs that locals and high-skilled talent would not consider. Singapore makes a concerted effort to keep these migrant workers in the shadows, despite making up more than a third of the labour force. Most notably, they have been hidden away through the construction of compact migrant worker dormitories which, with their spatial limitations, were ripe environments for transmission during the COVID-19 pandemic (The Online Citizen, 2020), as discussed in the next chapter.

COSMOPOLITAN SINGAPORE

Yeoh (2006: 29) contends that the state subjugates this population to a transient existence, so that they can be repatriated easily in economic downturns. In economically better times, their labour has been welcomed to build the urban landscape of Singapore. Building the cosmopolitan global city has long been a part of the Singapore project. Lee Kuan Yew articulated it loud and clear when he said:

> Singapore has to be as cosmopolitan as other world class cities like New York and London... Singaporeans, if I can choose an analogy, we are the hard disk of a computer, the foreign talent are the megabytes you add to your storage capacity. So your computer never hangs because you got enormous storage capacity. (Channel News Asia, 2007)

This is an echo of a legacy he and his fellow founding fathers established much earlier on. S. Rajaratnam's 1972 address explicitly calls upon Singapore to embrace its destiny as a global city: "we draw sustenance not only from the region, but also from the international economic system to which as a global city we belong and which will be final arbiter of whether we prosper or decline" (*The Strait Times*, 1972).

However, as a global city, Singapore differs from many other global metropolises in some key respects. Yeoh (2004) argues that the Singapore cosmopolis is limited by compartmentalized ideas about culture and identity, constrained in particular by 4 M's and CMIO: The former refers to the rather doctrinal notions of multiracialism, multiculturalism, multilingualism, and multireligiosity, while the second refers to a society rigidly composed of Chinese, Malay, Indian, and Other Singaporeans in fixed proportions. These doctrines constrain the more fluid and intersectional identities that inevitably arise with the sort of transnational mobility that characterizes Singapore. Yeoh suggests that there are at least three ways immigrants are viewed, which limit cosmopolitanism in Singapore:

"looking up to them" (the colonial mentality that the White expatriate is always right); "looking down on them" (colonial notions of superiority and inferiority in the allocation of "3D" [dirty, dangerous and difficult] jobs to foreign manual workers); and "fear of them" (fear of their physical presence and their "taking our jobs, our children's places in schools, and marrying our daughters" which mirrors the colonial obsession with "sanitation", "moral hygiene" and "racial purity"). (Yeoh, 2004: 2441)

In the nation-building project that runs alongside its cosmopolitaniza-tion, being "Singaporean" has been "manufactured through a series of founding myths and shared experiences" (Mathews and Soon, 2015). The citizens of this "city-nation-state" are very conscious of and attached to their national identity, as is typical of tiny countries surrounded by larger and more powerful neighbours (Lee, 2007). According to Yeoh and Lin (2013) and Chong (2015), some Singaporeans have become concerned that newcomers—and, by definition, temporary workers—do not share the same degree of loyalty to Singapore and the same set of values and norms. Hence, from this anthropological point of view, the PAP's narra-tive of attracting global talents to win "the war for talent" has in fact heightened Singaporean fears of being undermined by foreigners in their midst.

Singapore's immigration policy regime has struggled with these diver-gent and even contradictory attitudes. Singaporeans need foreigners but fear them at a deep level. The government recognizes these public concerns and occasionally tightens its liberal immigration policy to give Singaporeans confidence that they are prioritized over foreigners. And yet the crux of the strategy—to leverage high- and low-skilled foreign labour for economic growth and global prestige—remains broadly unchanged. This is an unsustainable situation, which finds an analogy in the frog that is slowly boiled alive.

THE PAP GOVERNMENT'S PRAGMATISM

From the time of Singapore's independence, the People's Action Party (PAP) government's pragmatic—meaning "non-ideological"—approach has pervaded nearly every policy realm. To achieve its goals of maximizing economic and material benefits for its citizens, the government has had to make modifications not only to its policy agenda, but also its principles (Tan, 2018: 17). Lee Kuan Yew described members of his party as:

> pragmatists. We don't stick to any ideology. Does it work? Let's try it, and if it does work, fine, let's continue it. If it doesn't work, toss it out, try another one. We are not enamoured with any ideology. (BBC News, 2015)

This pragmatic approach to governance has become the government's modus operandi. In the domain of immigration, however, policies seem to have remained entrenched, stubbornly unchanging even as circumstances seem to demand it. To illustrate this, we will discuss three critical junctures: the "Great Recession" of 2007–2009, Singapore's 2011 General Elections, and the 2013 Population White Paper. We argue that this sequence of events has led to the progressive deterioration of Singaporeans' perceptions of foreigners, immigration, and, to some extent, the PAP's Singapore as a political idea.

THE GREAT RECESSION OF 2007–2009

From December 2007 to June 2009, the developed world underwent the deepest recession since the Great Depression of the 1930s. The "Great Recession"—as this was called—pervaded most aspects of economic life, with the labour variable taking a hard hit. Indeed, the job market inevitably crunched, and the number of visas issued for both high- and low-skilled migrants soon dropped. The most affected were migrants temporarily working in OECD countries. They experienced tightening of inflow controls and were incentivized to return to their home countries if or when unemployed (OECD, 2009).

Governments had the challenging task of finding the right equilibrium between protectionism and liberalization of the labour market. If policies were too loose, as recommended by neoliberals, then the public would become inclined to portray foreign workers as the root cause of their reduced well-being. If policies dogmatically followed the protectionist agenda, then countries would run the risk of forfeiting long-term objectives such as coping with an ageing population, economic growth, and knowledge and skills transfer through global talent flows. It was a complex dilemma. At the end, a consensus was reached not to limit trade relationships as was done in the Great Depression's aftermath, but to limit their intakes of migrants and regulate more tightly those already in the national territory (OECD, 2009). One of the few countries that did not arrive at this consensus was Singapore.

Singapore officially slid into recession during the second quarter of 2008, when its economy contracted by 5.7% of its GDP (Balakrishnan, 2008). But this did not last long. By the end of 2009, the mature Asian Tiger recovered and, by 2010, its GDP annual growth "skyrocketed" up to 14.5% (World Bank, 2020). In Singapore, the Great Recession was an exogenous economic shock that occurred due to tight links with the West, particularly the United States. The vector for the economic contagion was the export-driven relationship with Western developed economies. Indeed, the city-state's exposure to external markets (Feenstra et al., 2015) has always been one of its greatest strengths and yet also a major vulnerability (Schwab, 2019: 19).

With a crunch in global demand, the economic consequences resonated extensively in Singapore's economy while its labour productivity declined to −6.5% in 2008 (Thangavelu, 2008). This decline in efficiency was due not only to economic shocks as firms came under pressure, but also to existing labour market structures. An excessive dependence on foreign workers, developed since the 1980s, had undermined the economy in terms of productivity (Barta and Venkat, 2010). Over the years, even though the PAP leadership has constantly promoted retraining and upskilling for a competitive national workforce that is ready for a "high-tech" era (Barry, 1986), the desired increase in productivity has not fully materialized. Indeed, as the government introduced more lenient immigration policies for specific categories of workers and allowed in a large number of low-skilled and low-waged migrant workers, there was little incentive for local businesses to take structural measures necessary for transforming the workforce to meet the new demands of the world economy. Such measures would have included the extension of training and reskilling or upskilling programmes. Lenient immigration policies also reduced the incentive for small and medium enterprises to invest in substantial improvements to their productive processes as cheap foreign labour abounded (Low et al., 2013).

So, when the Great Recession hit, the MOM and Workforce Development Agency (WDA) developed a more systemic retraining programme, called the Skills Programme for Upgrading and Resilience (SPUR), for Singaporeans who had been fired or suspended. In his speech at

Paradigma 2009—an event aimed at engaging Singaporean youth to act for social paradigm shift (Paradigma, 2010)—the former Minister for Manpower Gan Kim Yong (2009) explained clearly why the PAP changed its approach:

> *Singapore's only resource* lies in *our human capital.* We will nurture our own to be the best and brightest. At the same time, we also need to attract and retain good people from all around the world. Hence, we should welcome foreigners in Singapore [...] If we turf out the foreigners during the recession, we will be sending a wrong signal. Many of them will not return when we need them again after the recession is over. We need to adopt a balanced approach. As we continue to allow *calibrated access to foreign manpower*, we *must help Singaporeans* cope with the challenges. This, we have done through the Skills Programme for Upgrading and Resilience, or SPUR. (Emphasis added)

Gan acknowledged the necessity of pursuing a "balanced approach" to the workforce, and yet Singapore citizens perceived that not enough had been done to preserve their interests.

Control of the narrative is important as effective politics are hedged on communication and public perception (Herbert, 1969: 255). In the case of Singapore, which the 2020 Freedom House Index describes as only "partly free", the public response has been less reactive than in other democratic countries as it has been indoctrinated by years of government propaganda. Koh and colleagues (2017: 11) show how, between 2006 and 2014, no less than 80% of citizens were satisfied with the way their democratic system has been working. The PAP had been able to follow its long-term strategy as long as it could deliver economic and material benefit to the population, which also has the effect of numbing civic engagement in modern Singapore. Consequently, it now takes much more time before public discontent builds up and is openly voiced. The financial crisis triggered Singapore citizens to realize how much immigration policy had affected them and how it would continue to impact their lives in the years ahead.

In the aftermath of the global financial crisis, Singapore continued along the trajectory of its "pragmatic" neoliberal approach, pursuing an agenda of economic growth and material well-being through a reliance on foreign labour. Thus, many Singaporeans perceived immigration policy as too foreigner-friendly. A 2009 survey found a third of Singaporean youth, aged 21–29 years, feeling "worse off" by having to face foreign competition in the job market (Institute of Policy Studies, 2009: 8). Singapore's economic performance, it was felt, was no longer the means for achieving the well-being of its citizens and solving their bread-and-butter issues, but it had become the end of every government policy. Year after year, public discontent pertaining to inequality and working conditions in the job market grew, eroding the legitimacy of the PAP government.

By the end of the decade, the PAP government had increased the intake of foreigners as a response to the Great Recession. Its pragmatic neoliberal doctrine survived the global financial crisis and, in some respects, tightened its grip. Meanwhile the social compact between society and state weakened. Political opposition parties such as the Workers' Party and the Singapore Democratic Alliance picked up on this public dissatisfaction and made it one of the key issues in the 2011 General Elections.

THE GENERAL ELECTIONS OF 2011

Like GE2020 discussed in the previous chapter, Singapore's parliamentary elections in 2011—or GE2011—have often been described as a "watershed election", mainly because the PAP had their worst performance in history (Goh and Lee, 2011). It garnered "only" 60.1% of the popular vote. The opposition Workers' Party, on the other hand, obtained one of its best results with 39.9% of the total votes (Woon, 2017).

Scholars described this as a "new normal", when the electorate expressed fearlessly its discontent with the PAP's policies (Chong, 2012; Tan, 2012; Low, 2014). This was particularly true in respect of its liberal immigration policies. Singaporeans believed that income inequality and loss of their purchasing power in one of the most expensive cities in the world were only the tip of the iceberg.

In the aftermath of GE2011, then-Minister Mentor Lee Kuan Yew and then-Senior Minister Goh Chok Tong decided to retire from the new cabinet as they acknowledged in a joint statement that:

> The time has come for a younger generation [of PAP leaders] to carry Singapore forward in a more difficult and complex situation. [...] A *younger generation* [of citizens], besides having a non-corrupt and meritocratic government and a high standard of living, *wants to be more engaged* in the decisions which affect them. [...] But the younger team [of Cabinet

Ministers] must always have in mind *the interests of the older generation* [of citizens and PAP leaders]. (Quoted in Chang, 2011, Emphasis added)

In his 2011 National Day Rally speech, Prime Minister Lee Hsien Loong provided an analysis of what he thought were the key issues fought over in GE2011. These included public housing, public transport, inflation, and immigration. These concerns were confirmed by surveys in 2011 by the Institute of Policy Studies (IPS) and BlackBox Research. The IPS study concluded that a large proportion of the electorate "were younger and/or first-time voters" (IPS, 2011: 15) and 57% of respondents were worried about the influx of foreigners, which was one of the biggest concerns, second only to the rising cost of living (74%). In his speech, PM Lee addressed these issues extensively and he did so empathically. But when he considered the sensitive topic of immigration policy, he returned to a hardened PAP style, managing to echo once again many of its long-standing arguments about focusing on the long-term benefits to global-city Singapore of an open economy and society, and not to dwell on the immediate pains. Foreigners brought skills and added value to Singapore's benefit.

Subsequently, though, some immigration policies were revised. The criteria for obtaining certain passes were made more stringent. In between mid-2011 and 2013, at least three rounds of policy tightening were implemented for both high- and low-skilled workers (Yeoh and Lin, 2012). For example, since December 2011, foreign-born students studying in Singapore have only 3 months after graduation to look for a job and sign a contract, failing which they would be obliged to go back to their home countries. However, these revisions were really only cosmetic adjustments to soften Singaporeans on immigration matters. Where social cohesion was concerned, the government launched integration programmes to better engage new citizens "through home visits, grassroots activities, and community work [...], field trips to heritage sites, and community sharing" (Yeoh and Lin, 2012). While efforts had been in place, there was still a long way to success (Institute of Policy Studies, 2012).

THE POPULATION WHITE PAPER
AND LITTLE INDIA RIOT OF 2013

After GE2011, Singaporeans mostly welcomed the restrictive measures implemented on immigration inflows. However, when in 2013 the PAP government published its report titled "A Sustainable Population for a Dynamic Singapore", also known as the "Population White Paper" (PWP), Singaporeans were shocked and angered.

Due to Singapore's unfeasibly low total fertility rate, the PWP explained, its citizens would not be able to maintain a stable and sustainable population size in the years to come. Taking a pragmatic approach to the problem, the report openly praised all kinds of foreign workers as beneficial to the Singaporean economy, but at the same time recognized the need to limit the number of foreign workers coming in. Singaporeans have become accustomed to this style of narrative. So what made them angry this time was this point:

> By 2030, Singapore's total population could range between 6.5 and 6.9 million. [...] The resident population (comprising citizens and PRs) is projected to be 4.2 to 4.4 million, of which citizens alone will make up 3.6 to 3.8 million. (Government of Singapore, 2013a)

Singaporeans did the math and understood that this would mean that foreigners could make up 45% of the total population by 2030. During the parliamentary debate on the PWP, Prime Minister Lee gave a 90-minute speech showing, once again, his empathy with Singaporeans' concerns (Lim, 2013). He claimed that it was highly unlikely for the city-state's population to reach the 6.9 million number stated in the PWP, and that by 2030, no other increases were expected at all. The speech, like many others before, was designed to pacify an unhappy people who felt that their concerns had been ignored yet again. To the PAP's disappointment, this time it was not business-as-usual.

It took some Singaporeans less than a week to organize one of the largest demonstrations in the history of Singaporean dissent (Toh & AFP, 2013). More than 4,000 people gathered in Speakers' Corner to voice their discontent, a massive turnout by Singaporean protest standards (BBC, 2013). Gilbert Goh, one of the protest's organizers and GE2011 opposition candidate, told AFP reporters:

The large crowd here shows the PAP government that they [the protesters] *are not afraid anymore.* They don't want to hide behind a moniker on Facebook *to show their displeasure.* (BBC, 2013) (Emphasis added)

Criticisms did not only come from the public, but also from academics who considered the PWP's arguments "overly mechanistic, economically simplistic and astonishingly sociologically and politically naïve" (Tan, 2013).

On 8 December 2013, at the end of the year that began with the PWP's publication, a riot took place in Little India that left a deep scar on Singapore's collective memory. That evening, a bus ran over and killed an Indian migrant worker. This was the casus belli for a riot involving 400 men (CNA, 2013). Little India was the place at which many South Asian construction workers congregated on their weekend day off. In their ethnographic analysis, Hamid and Tutt (2019) note how the presence of these migrants was not always welcomed and local residents have complained about how "noisy and dirty" they were (Hamid and Tutt, 2019: 526). Singaporeans depend on migrant workers for the construction and maintenance of the global city. At the same time, anything more than the most basic instrumental view of their existence is seemingly unwelcomed. Many Singaporeans would prefer that these migrants be kept to the urban periphery, where most worker dormitories are now located.

The "Little India Riot"—as the incident has come to be known— created the conditions within which a moral panic could be observed, where "a condition, episode, person or group of persons emerges to become defined as a threat to societal values and interests" (Cohen, 2011: 1). It was not long before politically incorrect, xenophobic, and racist comments flooded the Internet (Pang and Ng, 2016), generally claiming that the majority of migrant workers were somehow dangerous and ungrateful for what Singapore society had offered them. These migrant workers were turned into "folk devils" to be feared for the threat they presented to Singapore's society and way of life.

The government condemned the rioters. When addressing the root of the problem, it quickly shifted the focus from immigration policy to alcohol consumption (Government of Singapore, 2013b; CNA, 2013). The government turned Little India into a "liquor control zone", enforcing restrictions on alcohol sale and consumption at certain times and days of the week. While excessive consumption of alcohol almost certainly had a part to play in causing the riot, the government was keen to downplay other more structural factors such as the poor living and working conditions of migrant workers, inadequate integration of migrants into mainstream society, racism and xenophobia, and the possibility that its immigration policies were too liberal to be sustainable (Au, 2013).

This critical moment could have been an opportunity to transform the immigration system structurally and holistically into a more balanced and inclusive one, aimed at concomitantly improving the well-being of Singaporeans and foreign workers. And yet, even in 2020, Prime Minister Lee explained in the clearest accent of neoliberal globalization that:

> Singapore has succeeded by being an international hub, tapping talents worldwide, and serving a global market. So even as we adjust our work pass policies, we must be careful not to give the wrong impression that we are now closing up, and no longer welcoming foreigners. Such a reputation would do us great harm, and we have to watch this, because we are being watched. [...] And we have to do the right thing for ourselves, but we must also avoid sending the wrong signals to others. (Lee, 2020)

As former United States President John F. Kennedy said during his 1962 State of the Union Address: "The time to repair the roof is when the sun is shining". Unfortunately, as the years passed and Singapore approached the early months of 2020, the sun had already set, and a thunderstorm was rolling in: the COVID-19 public health crisis came with strong implications for the immigration and economic agenda.

The Impact of the Pandemic
on Foreigners in Singapore

Although the Singapore government's immigration policy has been a lot more liberal than many Singaporeans are comfortable with, the COVID-19 pandemic has been challenging for foreigners in Singapore. Large numbers of expatriates have been stranded abroad, unable to enter Singapore to take up the jobs that they had accepted, even with visas in hand. Many have been afraid of leaving the country as they may not be allowed to return (Aravindan and Chen, 2021). Many feel that the border restrictions and vaccination eligibility criteria, which are different for citizens and foreigners, are simply unfair. These expatriate pandemic experiences are not unique to Singapore, but they do contrast sharply with the foreigner-friendly experience they had enjoyed before COVID-19 created tension between keeping the economy open, protecting Singaporeans from infection and harm, and minimizing citizens' unhappiness including their feelings of betrayal so that they will continue to support the PAP establishment.

To find a new balance, the government started another cycle of tightening its policies on giving employment priority to Singaporeans over foreigners, in no small part a response to rising popular and party-political pressure as the local middle class is increasingly confronted by the longer-term trend of technological change and the sudden impact of a pandemic, both utterly disruptive to their job prospects and livelihoods.

Badly behaving expats regularly feature in the mainstream media and attract much anger and frustration from local netizens, as well as foreign ones embarrassed by such behaviour. During the pandemic, foreigners who openly flouted the safe management measures in public were not spared. The government revoked the employment passes of expats who disregarded the circuit-breaker restrictions. It also deported a British man for refusing to wear a mask while travelling in public transport (Silver, 2021).

As more Singaporeans, provoked by the challenges of the pandemic, feel left behind, the ground will become more fertile for authoritarian-populist politics. Foreigners are usually the first to be targeted, followed by the technocratic establishment whose policies seem to favour them. Meanwhile, the government, still wedded to the belief that foreign talent is crucial for Singapore's survival and success, makes concessionary shifts in ways that attempt to signal empathy and responsiveness to Singaporeans, while continuing to make welcoming overtures to foreign professionals.

The next chapter discusses the impact of the pandemic on the working-class group of migrants, qualitatively different from the problems that expats have faced in Singapore and certainly more challenging.

REFERENCES

Aravindan, A., & Chen, L. (2021). Expats wait anxiously as Singapore weighs COVID-19 reopening. Reuters, 6 August.

Au, A. (2013, 10 December). Riot in Little India: Spark and fuel. Yawning Bread. https://yawningbread.wordpress.com/2013/12/10/riot-in-little-india-spark-and-fuel/. Accessed 15 November 2020.

Balakrishnan, A. (2008). Singapore slides into recession. *The Guardian.* https://www.theguardian.com/business/2008/oct/10/creditcrunch-market turmoil1. Accessed 20 November 2020.

Barry, W. (1986). Human resources in Singapore's second industrial revolution. *Industrial Relations Journal, 17(2),* 99–114. https://doi.org/10.1111/j.1468-2338.1986.tb00529.x.

Barta, P., & Venkat, P. R. (2010). Singapore moves to curtail immigration. *Wall Street Journal.* https://www.wsj.com/articles/SB1000142405274870 34944045750813029415754 36. Accessed 20 November 2020.

BBC News. (2013). Rare mass rally over Singapore immigration plan [online] bbc.com. Available at: https://www.bbc.com/news/world-asia-21485729. Accessed 20 October 2020.

BBC News. (2015, 22 March). *In quotes: Lee Kuan Yew.* London: BBC. https://www.bbc.com/news/world-asia-31582842. Accessed 20 November 2020.

Chang, R. (2011, 15 May). MM Lee, SM Goh to retire from Cabinet. *The Straits Times.* https://www.straitstimes.com/GeneralElection/News/Story/STIStory_668597.html. Accessed 20 November 2020.

Chong, T. (2012). A return to normal politics: Singapore general elections 2011. *Southeast Asian Affairs,* vol. 2012, 283–298.

Chong, T. (2015). Stepping stone Singapore: The cultural politics of anti-immigrant anxieties. In Yap Mui Teng, Gillian Koh & Debbie Soon (Eds.), *Migration and integration in Singapore: Policies and practice* (pp. 214–229). London: Routledge.

CNA. (2013, 22 December). Spotlight: A look back at Singapore's first riot in more than 40 years [video] YouTube. Available at https://www.youtube.com/watch?v=X_rypQ8vXXU. Accessed 19 October 2020.

Cohen, S. (2011). *Folk devils and moral panics* (3rd ed.). London: Routledge classics.

Department of Statistics. (2020). Labour market report advance release second quarter 2020.

Dobbs, S., & Loh, K. S. (2019). Open or bordered? Singapore, industrialisation and Malaysian workers. *Asian Studies Review, 43(2),* 206–223. https://doi.org/10.1080/10357823.2019.1590312.

Feenstra, R. C., Inklaar, R., & Timmer, M. P. (2015). The next generation of the penn world table. *American Economic Review, 105(10),* 3150–3182.

Freedom House. (2020). Singapore. Freedom House. https://freedomhouse.org/country/singapore/freedom-world/2020. Accessed 20 November 2020.

Goh, C. T., & Lee, K. Y. (2011). Joint statement of Mentor Minister Lee and Senior Minister Goh. Reproduced in R. Chang (Ed.), MM Lee, SM Goh to retire from Cabinet *The Straits Times*. https://web.archive.org/web/201 10516065503/http://www.straitstimes.com/GeneralElection/News/Story/ STIStory_668597.html. Accessed 20 November 2020.

Gan, Kim Yong (2009). Speech at paradigma 2009—Going beyond the global financial crisis: Thoughts & reflections. Ministry of Manpower. https://www. mom.gov.sg/newsroom/speeches/2009/speech-by-mr-gan-kim-yong-min ister--at-the-paradigma-2009--going-beyond-the-global-financial-crisis-tho ughts--reflections-15-july-2009-210-pm-anderson-junior-college.   Accessed 10 November 2020.

Government of Singapore. (2013a). A sustainable population for a dynamic Singapore: Population white paper. https://raw.githubusercontent.com/iso merpages/isomerpages-stratgroup/master/images/PublicationImages/cha rt7.png.pdf. Accessed 20 November 2020.

Government of Singapore. (2013b). What are the facts of the rioting incident at Little India on 8 Dec? https://www.gov.sg/article/what-are-the-facts-of-the-rioting-incident-at-little-india-on-8-dec. Accessed 15 November 2020.

Government of Singapore. (2020). Why do we need skilled foreign workers in Singapore? 6 July. https://www.gov.sg/article/why-do-we-need-skilled-for eign-workers-in-singapore. Accessed 20 November 2020.

Hamid, W., & Tutt, D. (2019). Thrown away like a banana leaf: Precarity of labour and precarity of place for Tamil migrant construction workers in Singa pore. *Construction Management and Economics, 37*(9), 513–536 (2019). https://doi.org/10.1080/01446193.2019.1595075.

Herbert, E. A. (1969). Communications and politics: The media and the message. *Law and Contemporary Problems, 34*, 255–277. https://scholarship. law.duke.edu/lcp/vol34/iss2/4. Accessed 20 November 2020.

HSBC. (2020). Expat explorer: Broadening perspectives. https://www.expatexpl orer.hsbc.com/global-report/. Accessed 8 May 2021.

Humanitarian Organization for Migration Economics (HOME). (2017). No privacy, no space: Domestic workers endure poor living condi tions. https://www.home.org.sg/our-updates/2017/11/30/no-privacy-no-space-domestic-workers-endure-poor-living-conditions. Accessed May 9 2021.

Institute of Policy Studies. (2009). Resilience in the economic crisis. National University of Singapore, *POPS* (1), 13. https://lkyspp.nus.edu.sg/docs/def ault-source/ips/pops-1_report_0209.pdf. Accessed 20 November 2020.

Institute of Policy Studies. (2011). IPS post-election forum. National University of Singapore, *POPS* (4), 25. https://lkyspp.nus.edu.sg/docs/default-source/ ips/pops-4_report_0511.pdf. Accessed 20 November 2020.

Institute of Policy Studies. (2012). Conference on integration. IPS social markers of integration survey, National University of Singa pore. https://lkyspp.nus.edu.sg/docs/default-source/ips/SI_S2_Dr-Leong-Chan-Hoong_2205.pdf. Accessed 20 November 2020.

Kennedy, J. F. (1962). State of the Union Address, 11 January 1962 [Reel 1]. John F. Kennedy Presidential Library and Museum. https://www.jfklibrary. org/asset-viewer/archives/JFKWHA/1962/JFKWHA-066/JFKWHA-066. Accessed 20 November 2020.

Kerr, S. P., Kerr, W., Özden, Ç., & Parsons, C. (2016). Global talent flows. *Journal of Economic Perspectives, 30* (4), 83–106.

Koh, G., Tan, E. S., & Soon, D. (2017). Asian Barometer country report— Singapore. ABS Working Paper Series 147, 35. http://asianbarometer.org/ publications/abs-working-paper-series. Accessed 20 November 2020.

Lee, H. L. (2007). Parliamentary debate on Civil Service salary revisions. https://www.nas.gov.sg/archivesonline/data/pdfdoc/20070411980. htm. Accessed 20 November 2020.

Lee, H. L. (2011). National Day Rally 2011. Prime Minister's Office, Government of Singapore. https://www.pmo.gov.sg/Newsroom/prime-minister-lee-hsien-loongs-national-day-rally-2011-speech-english. Accessed 19 October 2020.

Lee, H. L. (2020). Transcript of PM Lee Hsien Loong's speech at the debate on the motion of thanks to the President on 2 September 2020. Prime Minister's Office, Government of Singapore. https://www.pmo.gov.sg/New sroom/PM-Lee-Speech-at-the-debate-on-the-motion-of-thanks-to-the-presid ent-Sep-2020. Accessed 30 October 2020.

Lee, K. Y. (1959). Speech by the Prime Minister at the Official Opening of the Civil Service Study Centre, 15 August.

Lim, L. (2013). Parliament endorses population white paper by a vote of 77 to 13. *The Straits Times.* https://www.straitstimes.com/singapore/parliament-endorses-population-white-paper-by-a-vote-of-77-to-13. Accessed 25 October 2020.

Low, L. (2002). The political economy of migrant worker policy in Singapore. *Asia Pacific Business Review, 8*(4), 95–118 (2002). https://doi.org/ 10.1080/713999166.

Low, D., Yeoh, L. K., Tan, K. S., & Bhaskaran, M. (2013). *IPS Commons.* Research Collection School Of Economics.

Low, D. (2014). Governing in the new normal. In D. Low & S. T. Vadaketh (Ed.), *Hard choices: Challenging the Singapore consensus.* Singapore: National University Press.

Mathews, M., & Soon, D. (2015). Transiting into the Singaporean identity: Immigration and naturalisation policy. *Migration Letters, 13*(1), 33–48.

Ministry of Manpower. (1999). *Manpower21: Vision of a talent capital.* Singapore: MOM.

Ministry of Manpower. (2018). Foreign worker experience survey, 2018. Government of Singapore. https://www.mom.gov.sg/-/media/mom/documents/ statistics-publications/foreign-worker-study-2011.pdf. Accessed 23 October 2020.

Ministry of Manpower. (2020). Foreign workforce numbers. Government of Singapore. http://www.mom.gov.sg/documents-and-publications/foreign-workforce-numbers. Accessed 24 October 2020.

Migration Policy Institute. (2012). Rapid growth in Singapore's immigrant population brings policy challenges. https://www.migrationpolicy.org/article/rapid-growth-singapores-immigrant-population-brings-policy-challenges. Accessed 2 November 2020.

OECD. (2009). International migration: Charting a course through the crisis. Policy Brief. OECD. http://www.oecd.org/migration/mig/International%20Migration%20Charting%20a%20course%20through%20the%20crisis.pdf. Accessed 15 October 2020.

Pang, N., & Ng, J. (2016). Twittering the Little India Riot: Audience responses, information behavior and the use of emotive cues. *Computers in Human Behavior, 54*, 607–619 (2016). https://doi.org/10.1016/j.chb.2015.08.047.

Paradigma. (2010). What is Paradigma? PARADIGMA 2010. https://paradigma2010.wordpress.com/what-is-paradigma/. Accessed 25 November 2020.

Paul, A. M., & Long, V. (2016). Human-capital strategies to build world-class research universities in Asia: Impact on global flows. In M. H. Chou, I. Kamola, & T. Pietsch (Eds.), *Transnational politics of higher education: Contesting the global/transforming the local* (pp. 130–155) Abingdon: Routledge.

Poh, Madeleine. (2016). Analysing the recent changes to legislation surrounding foreign domestic workers in Singapore. *Singapore Law Review.* http://www.singaporelawreview.com/juris-illuminae-entries/tag/Madeleine+Poh. Accessed 25 October 2020.

Schwab, K. (2019). The global competitiveness report 2019. Insight report. World Economic Forum. http://www3.weforum.org/docs/WEF_TheGlobalCompetitivenessReport2019.pdf.

Sidhu, R., Ho, K. C., & Yeoh, B. (2010). Emerging education hubs: The case of Singapore. *Higher Education, 61*(1), 23–40 (2011). https://doi.org/10.1007/s10734-010-9323-9.

Sidhu, R., Ho, K. C., & Yeoh, B. S. A. (2011). The global schoolhouse: Governing Singapore's knowledge economy aspirations. In S. Marginson, S. Kaur, & E. Sawir (Eds.), *Higher education in the Asia-Pacific* (pp. 255–271). Dordrecht: Springer.

Silver, K. (2021). COVID threatens Singapore's business hub crown. *BBC News,* 31 August.

Tan, J. (2013). Population white paper triggers nationwide debate. Yahoo! News. https://sg.news.yahoo.com/-yir2013--population-white-paper-triggers-nationwide-debate-101840966.html. Accessed 24 October 2020.

Tan, K. P. (2012). Singapore in 2011. *Asian Survey, 52*(1), 220–226 (2001). https://doi.org/10.1525/as.2012.52.1.220.

Tan, K. P. (2018). *Singapore: Identity, brand, power.* Cambridge (UK): Cambridge University Press.

Teo, T. (2019). *Civic multiculturalism in Singapore: Revisiting citizenship, rights and recognition.* Cham: Springer International Publishing. https://doi.org/10.1007/978-3-030-13459-4.

Thangavelu, S. M. (2008). Global financial crisis: Impact on Singapore and ASEAN. EABER Working Papers. East Asian Bureau of Economic Research. The Australian National University. Accessed 2 October 2020.

The ASEAN Post. (2020, May 3) Why Singapore turns to foreign talent. *The ASEAN Post.* https://theaseanpost.com/article/why-singapore-turns-for eign-talent. Accessed 9 October 2020.

The Online Citizen. (2020, 7 April). Condition of the migrant worker's dormitories nearly ideal for transmission of infection. https://www.onlinecit izenasia.com/2020/04/07/twc2-condition-of-the-migrant-workers-dormit ories-nearly-ideal-for-transmission-of-infection/.

The Straits Times. (1972, 7 February). 'Global city' success for Singapore: Raja. Page 1. Accessed from *NewspaperSG,* a Singapore Government Agency Website.

The Straits Times. (2020, 26 October). Veteran migrant workers: Singapore is land of opportunity. https://www.straitstimes.com/singapore/veteran-mig rant-workers-singapore-is-land-of-opportunity

Toh, H. S., & AFP. (2013). Singapore protest biggest since independence. *South China Morning Post.* https://www.scmp.com/news/asia/article/115 2046/singapore-protest-population-policy-biggest-independence. Accessed 20 October 2020.

Woon, C. Y. (2017). Internet spaces and the (re)making of democratic politics: The case of Singapore's 2011 General Election. *GeoJournal, 83,* 1133–1150 (2018). https://doi.org/10.1007/s10708-017-9815-6.

World Bank. (2020). GDP growth (annual %)—Singapore. The World Bank Data: Washington. https://data.worldbank.org/indicator/NY.GDP.MKTP. KD.ZG?locations=SG. Accessed 17 October 2020.

Yang, P. (2018). Desiring 'Foreign talent': Lack and Lacan in anti-immigrant sentiments in Singapore. *Journal of Ethnic and Migration Studies, 44*(6), 1015–1031 (2018). https://doi.org/10.1080/1369183X.2017.1384157.

Yeoh, B. S. A. (2004). Cosmopolitanism and its exclusions in Singapore. *Urban Studies, 41*(12), 2431–2445.

Yeoh, B. S. A. (2006). Bifurcated labour: The unequal incorporation of transmigrants in Singapore. *Tijdschrift voor Economische en Sociale Geografie, 97*(1), 26–37. https://doi.org/10.1111/j.1467-9663.2006.00493.x.

Yeoh, B. S. A., & Lin, W. (2012). Rapid growth in Singapore's immigration population brings policy challenges. Migration Policy Institute. https://www.migrationpolicy.org/article/rapid-growth-singapores-imm igrant-population-brings-policy-challenges. Accessed 19 October 2020.

Yeoh, B. S. A., & Lin, W. (2013). Chinese migration to Singapore: Discourses and discontents in a globalizing nation-state. *Asia and Pacific Migration Journal*, *22*(1), 31–53. https://doi.org/10.1177/011719681302200103.

CHAPTER 6

Migrant Worker Dormitories: Virus in a Neoliberal Politics of Space

Carolin Bernhard and Mara Ellemunt

Abstract In neoliberal Singapore, capitalism thrives on the exploitation of low-waged migrant workers who are attracted to Singapore to earn a living building and cleaning the city and serving its residents. Their presence in this already crowded city provokes a dualistic public response that originates from a grudging acceptance of their indispensability: on the one hand, a refusal to allow them to fully integrate with Singapore society and be treated as equal human beings; and, on the other hand, a compassionate desire to help them when they are in need. The former tendency has had the effect of making migrant workers as invisible as possible, hence the profitable solution to house large numbers of them in dormitories located in the peripheral spaces of the island. Capitalism,

C. Bernhard (✉)
Double Master Degree in Public Policy and European Affairs, National University of Singapore and Sciences Po (2021), Neustadt, Germany
e-mail: carolin.bernhard@u.nus.edu; carolin.bernhard@sciencespo.fr

M. Ellemunt
Double Master Degree in Public Policy and European Affairs, National University of Singapore and Sciences Po (2021), Perca, Italy
e-mail: ellemunt.mara@u.nus.edu; mara.ellemunt@sciencespo.fr

© The Author(s), under exclusive license to Springer Nature
Singapore Pte Ltd. 2022
K. P. Tan (ed.), *Singapore's First Year of COVID-19*,
https://doi.org/10.1007/978-981-19-0368-7_6

profit maximization, and space optimization have created conditions and practices of exploitation that are, in normal times, cloaked in invisibility. The 2020 outbreak of COVID-19 in these dormitory spaces should not be surprising, unless they had been so well-hidden in the blind spots of public conscience and policy consciousness. The outbreaks also produced dualistic public reactions: moral panic and the stigmatization of infectious foreigners as dirty and dangerous folk devils, which demands further spatial segregation; and civic activism that steps up to the service of helping the vulnerable in their time of need. The solutions going forward will likely be technical rather than normative in nature, well within the segregating and exploitative logic of neoliberal globalization, with ever-more-ingenious ways to extract value from migrant-worker labour, while making them and the heterotopia in which they exist as invisible and distant as possible.

Keywords Migrant workers · Dormitories · Stigmatization · Moral panic · Spatial segregation · Heterotopia · Civic activism

A "Pandemic of Inequality" (Tan, 2020) was the headline of a BBC news report on COVID-19 in Singapore. By late October 2020, 10 months after the first COVID-19 case had been reported on the island-state, nearly 95% of almost 60,000 total infections at the time occurred in migrant worker dormitories (MOH, 2020). While the rapid virus spread in densely populated communities with high rates of social interactions is a non-normative scientific fact (Hamidi et al., 2020), state policy responses to the pandemic outbreak in the dormitories invite closer scrutiny of underlying normative political decisions, economic interests, and social pressures linked to virus containment.

Tracing the COVID-19 spread in Singapore's migrant worker dormitories, this chapter puts forward a theory- and policy-informed framework to analyze the pandemic in the context of how migrant workers are understood and managed in Singapore. In particular, their dormitories are spaces of political, social, and economic contestation, encapsulating the dynamics of neoliberal globalization and practices of spatial segregation. Beyond simply revealing the poor living conditions that migrant workers are subjected to in dormitories, COVID-19 highlights their precarity in a highly lucrative labour migration business in Singapore. The virus also makes clear a contradiction within the wider public, which leads to stigmatisation and discrimination on the one hand, but also empathy and solidarity with the migrant worker community on the other.

Migrant Workers and the Precarity of Place

The number of low-waged migrant workers has grown rapidly over the past twenty years, enabling Singapore's hyper-modernisation, including numerous large-scale infrastructure projects. Out of the current total foreign workforce of approximately 1.3 million, more than 940,000 workers are semi-skilled Work Permit holders (MOM, 2020b). Over half of them pursued secondary education in their countries of departure. Ten per cent obtained university education (Fordyce, 2020). And yet, the prospect of better living conditions and higher incomes compared to their country-of-origin are key pull factors for migrating to Singapore to take up jobs for which they seem overqualified. Notably, the majority of low-waged female migrant workers take on roles as live-in domestic workers in Singapore. A large share of the male migrant population finds employment in construction, marine shipyard, and process (CMP) sectors, while living in different types of shared accommodations (TWC2, 2020c). This chapter mainly focuses on these low-waged construction workers (hereafter "migrant workers"), predominantly coming from countries across South Asia including India and Bangladesh, China, Thailand, and the Philippines.

CMP workers engage in so-called 3D-work that is deemed "dangerous, dirty and degrading" (Chin, 2019). As part of a "low-cost, hyper-productive, docile and disposable" labour force, they are constantly exposed to various forms of precarity (Baey and Yeoh, 2015: 12). Indeed, "precarity is symptomatic of the socially 'corrosive' effects of neoliberal capitalism", as Singaporean sociologists Grace Baey and Brenda Yeoh (2018: 252) observe. In the context of migrant worker employment, such corrosion materialises at all stages of the labour migration process. From the very start of their labour migration pathway, many migrants enter vicious cycles of indebtedness vis-à-vis local brokers and job agents, who macro-manage various job placements (Wee et al., 2018). Singaporean NGOs that support migrant workers, such as the Humanitarian Organisation for Migration Economics (HOME), report debt levels of US$6,000 to US$7,000 (Wham, 2020). The organization Transient Workers Count Too (TWC2) estimates first-time recruitment fees of up to US$15,000

(Fordyce, 2020). Such high levels of indebtedness in turn make migrant workers all the more compliant to tolerate precarious work and life conditions (Wham, 2020).

The legal status of many migrant workers in Singapore is highly contingent on employer-sponsored Work Permits (Chok, 2017). This dependency on employers subsequently translates into entrapment in oftentimes exploitative, non-amendable contracts. Inflexible working arrangements and the absence of job security due to temporary employment arrangements further underpin their precarity. In sum, such employment schemes essentially leave low-waged migrant workers "at the bottom of neoliberal capitalist labour markets" (Baey and Yeoh, 2018: 249).

Within Singapore's migration management system—a complex network of state regulations and market forces—private employers and NGO activists all play a part in shaping migrant workers' subjective experiences of precarity, its exacerbation on the one hand and potential mitigation on the other. While their postings at CMP sites entail numerous risks in terms of dangerous work conditions and potential accidents, financial and language barriers hinder the access to basic healthcare services and post-injury medical treatment (Ang et al., 2019; Lee et al., 2014).

Beyond the realm of work, precarity is equally tied to social spaces and life design. As Brett Neilson and Ned Rossiter (2006: 10) explain:

> Precarity leads to an interminable lack of certainty, the condition of being unable to predict one's fate or having some degree of stability on which to construct a life that extends beyond the world of work to encompass other aspects of intersubjective life, including housing, debt and the ability to build affective social relations.

Migrant worker dormitories exemplify a "precarity of place". The concept has been theorized by Australian sociologist Susan Banki (2013), who studied Burmese migrant workers in Thailand. Banki describes precarity of place as a lack of individual autonomy, which is heavily regulated and shaped by state policies and regulations (Hamid and Tutt, 2019). Dormitory arrangements in the Singapore context have created precarious health conditions in which infectious diseases may spread easily and uncontrollably (Sadarangani et al., 2017). Yet, closely interlinked with non-normative biological and public health-related concerns are numerous biopolitical as much as societal considerations, which ultimately underpin the dormitories' nature as sites of political contestation, including the generation of precarity and social exclusion.

Migrant Worker Dormitories: Heterotopia and Moral Panic

The rapid spread of COVID-19 in migrant worker dormitories has critically revealed longstanding precarious housing conditions, linked to poor sanitation and limited space (Ratcliffe, 2020), while further exacerbating migrants' precarity of place. In the context of migrant workers' accommodation management, precarious spaces are formed by the host government's policies and practices that create an "absence of the permission to live freely and securely in one's physical place". Simultaneously, the dormitories as precarious spaces confront migrant workers with the expression of exclusionary social practices in their everyday experience in Singapore (Hamid and Tutt, 2019: 522). Singapore's neoliberal management of migrant workers implies the "national assignment of privileges and benefits". Privileges and benefits are allocated to segments of society that are concentrated within certain physical spaces. Correspondingly, Singapore's management of migrant workers and the precarity of place reflects the absence of such privileges and benefits, for instance the permission to move freely in space or the vulnerability of being deported (Banki, 2013).

Space has always been a sensitive topic for Singapore, reflected in the city-state's self-perceived vulnerability and deeply grounded in its siege mentality as discussed in Chapter 2. With the development of Singapore's economy, the government took firm control over its scarce space with the aim of optimizing its functional efficiency to ensure wealth accumulation within a capitalist society (Zieleniec, 2007). Hence, the control of space is political control in the name of economic growth. Being political, it entails simultaneously social control, exercised by the government over its population, resulting in socio-spatial exclusion for migrant workers (Sibley, 1995). The capitalist depiction of space turned it into a means of production and an object of consumption. Space is perceived and used like a machine with the aim of generating outcomes, which can either be understood in social or economic terms. The social and economic outcomes of space as a means of production is ultimately generated by the spatial arrangement, such as the decision to concentrate dormitories or aggregate industry (Lefebvre, 2009). The competition for space is especially pressing in the face of scarcity, leading to urban strategies of space maximization. Indeed, space in Singapore has become a precious social and political commodity, tied to specific purposes and goals (Lefebvre, 2009). Beyond rigorous urban planning, the social component, that again is attributed to space through its control, amplifies already existing spatial segregation. The perpetuation of this segregation exacerbates inequalities and finally creates new conglomerates of spaces within the city. More than 40 migrant worker dormitories, licensed in accordance with the Foreign Employee Dormitory Act (FEDA), are concentrated in the island's peripheral spaces as clear examples of spatial segregation.

In other words, migrant dormitories are a manifestation of space maximization within a competitive capitalist environment. The majority of Singapore's migrant construction workers, who number around 200,000, are housed in 43 licensed purpose-built dormitories (PBDs) with capacities between 3,000 and 25,000 workers each. Typically, 12–20 workers occupy one room and share sanitary and recreational facilities (Chin et al., 2020). FEDA regulates standards of living and prescribes a minimum space of 4.5 m^2 per worker as well as contingency plans. Despite regulations and high fines of up to $50,000, the Ministry of Manpower (MOM) reported non-compliance of around 20 PBDs in 2020 (Sen and Ong, 2020; MOM, 2020a).

These requirements do not apply to other housing, such as the 1,200 factory-converted dormitories (FCDs) and temporary quarters in construction sites. The former house 95,000 workers and the latter another 20,000 workers. Another 85,000 workers are either accommodated in Housing and Development Board (HDB) flats, condominiums, or private premises (Sen and Ong, 2020). FCDs are considered as independent workers' dormitories within industrial or warehouse developments. Due to this classification, FCDs require approval from the Urban Redevelopment Authority (URA), as opposed to temporary quarters that fall under the regulations of the Building and Construction Authority (BCA) and MOM. Unlike PBDs, these housing sites are not regulated by the FEDA. However, URA guidelines propose a minimum living standard of 4.5 m^2 per resident. In private premises, up to six workers can be housed in each unit, regardless of its size (MOM, 2020c). The numerous dormitories that are not regulated under FEDA and URA guidelines suffer from excessive space "optimization", concentrating a large number of workers in each of these places.

In these migrant worker dormitory spaces, the formal division of responsibilities among the authorities, dormitory operators, employers, and migrant workers is blurred. Within their administrative ambiguity, there is lack of ownership of arising problems. Migrant workers may be confused or uncertain about their rights, liabilities, or even contact persons in case of emergencies. According to the Employment of Foreign Manpower (Work Passes) Regulations 2012, employers must assume the responsibility for their workers including food, medical treatment, and housing. However, they are not empowered to directly influence the housing conditions, such as the number of people who can stay in one room or the level of cleanliness. Dormitory operators administer the dormitories and are in charge of upkeeping their conditions, while meeting the respective requirements that are dictated by the authorities. Yet, as the case discussion of COVID-19 in the dormitories will show, the blurring of responsibilities between employers and dormitory operators became obvious during the pandemic. MOM shifted the responsibility for housing conditions to the employers by advising them to ensure that their work pass holders "are observing... safe distancing measures" while penalizing "irresponsible practices and behavior" (Loong, 2020).

Both spatial segregation and the dormitories' complex management dynamics have in many ways created structural barriers for public engagement and information exchange, thereby feeding into the perception of dormitories as contested places of "the other"—a so-called heterotopia. Michel Foucault conceptualized a heterotopia as a real place of "the different", as opposed to an unreal space of utopia (Foucault, 1984). Olga Lafazani (2013) uses the Foucauldian notion of heterotopia in the context of migration. She applies it to migrants' squatter settlements, depicting them as isolated spaces, with a certain function of hosting the other. Foucault's heterotopia of deviation describes places "in which individuals whose behaviour is deviant in relation to the required mean or norm are placed" (Foucault, 1984). Deviation might also consist in projected behaviours that often respond to given stereotypes of "the other" within the host society. Erich Goode and Nachman Ben-Yahuda (2009) link the unknown and fear of deviance, that is often perceived as violation of a society's norms or rules, to moral panics. Indeed, deviance is a source of moral panics that is primarily defined by the audience that experiences or hears about it and subsequently evaluates it, rather than by the behaviour or belief per se. Migrant worker dormitories can thus be considered a space of the other and source of moral panics within the Singaporean city.

PUBLIC DISCOURSE: US VS. THEM

Whether conceived in terms of socio-economic or cultural similarities and differences, the notion of the "other" allows for the construction of imagined communities (Anderson, 1983). In treating migrant workers as part of a floating "out-group", some Singaporeans have behaved in ways that foster exclusion and stigmatisation, driven by the prejudice of a self-declared, albeit heterogeneous, "in-group" (Allport, 1954). Especially where migrant worker dormitories are concerned, these attitudes resonate with David Sibley's (1995) concept of geographies of exclusion. The concept refers to ways of socio-spatial exclusion, signalling unwelcome towards minorities. In Sibley's terms, migrant workers can be depicted as disorderly and needing to be policed and supervised. This, in turn, creates the conditions for moral panic to emerge.

A study by the International Labour Organization (2019) surveyed a sample of 1,005 Singaporeans on their attitudes towards migrant workers, including foreign domestic workers and construction workers. While 58% of respondents acknowledged the positive effect of migrant workers on the economy and the need for more low-skilled workers, 60% believed that migrant workers should not receive the same benefits and salary as local workers, while 36% believed that migrant workers should not receive equal working conditions as locals.

Worried about shrinking asset values, as well as perceived threats associated with migrant workers, such as crime, littering, and congestion, some Singaporeans have taken a "not-in-my-backyard" (NIMBY) attitude towards proposals to site foreign worker housing within their neighbourhood. The ILO (2019) study showed that 31% of Singaporean respondents (the highest percentage among the surveyed countries) agreed that migration negatively impacts crime rates. Furthermore, 32% believed migrant workers had poor work ethics and were untrustworthy, and 53% perceived them as a threat to Singapore's culture and heritage. Such underlying perceptions fuel populist rhetoric and moral panics. An actual panic is grounded in the de-facto threat posed by an event that is sustained by objective numbers and narratives. In contrast, moral panics are usually heightened actual panics that are disproportionate to the actual threat (Goode and Ben-Yahuda, 2009).

Characterizing migrant workers as potential criminals goes back to the 1980s, when then-Labour Minister S. Jayakumar claimed that "more migrant workers were involved in crimes such as shoplifting and fighting" (The Straits Times, 1983). At the time, the government aimed to reduce their number due to increased immigration offenses in the construction industry. In 2008, in the context of a NIMBY campaign, the police tried to moderate public resistance against the building of a migrant worker dormitory in the Serangoon Gardens neighbourhood by officially stating that "temporary migrant workers have a lower rate of arrest compared to Singaporeans and that they are largely law-abiding". This incident demonstrates how perceived threat and actual moral panics might diverge (Bal, 2017). Indeed, detention rates in 2018 largely confirm this discrepancy, with 4,489 foreigners arrested as opposed to 12,731 Singaporeans and permanent residents (Singapore Government, 2020a).

Traditional and social media discourse present multiple narratives regarding migrant worker issues in Singapore. Within a spectrum of opinions and attitudes, a common thread is the differentiation between the community and migrant workers. According to Duttaand his colleagues (2016), the media coverage of the Little India riots, following a migrant worker's fatal death in a bus accident in 2013, was based on stigmatization and the exoticization of migrant workers, creating a narrative of migrants behaving differently. Official explanations of the Little India riots cast the migrant workers' behaviour as almost entirely cultural, linked to the consumption of alcohol and street justice as "a trait of Indian culture". This assessment led to the introduction of limits on alcohol sale and consumption in public places, as well as the installation of more street lighting and surveillance cameras (Sim and Kok 2015). To put more distance between migrant workers and mainstream society, greater numbers of fenced up accommodation with self-contained recreational facilities were presented as a feasible solution (Goh, 2014). Sibley (1995) argues how, in geographies of exclusion, spatial boundaries are congruent with "moral boundaries". In the aftermath of Singapore's Little India riots, spatial boundaries were secured by attributing undesirable cultural traits to migrant workers through a certain type of public discourse that generated sharper moral boundaries.

Covid-19 in the Dormitories

At the time of the first migrant worker's COVID-19 infection in Singapore, the country's 42nd case announced on 9 February 2020, the government had laid out an effective pandemic management plan and succeeded in containing the virus spread through meticulous tracing, as discussed in Chapter 4. At a first emergency meeting on 25 to 26 January 2020, representatives from MOM and the Ministry of Health (MOH) had already discussed potential action plans for migrant worker dormitories, whereby "dormitory managers were told they need to prepare isolation rooms" for suspected or positive cases (Phua, 2020b). An advisory issued by MOM further called on the dormitory operators to prevent inter-mixing of residents between blocks and floors. During this pre-crisis phase, most decisions concerning virus containment in the dormitories and emergency plans thus remained under the dormitory operators' responsibility, beyond their function as mere landlords (Ling, 2020).

A false sense of security was fostered by the absence of immediate COVID-19 clusters arising from Case 42, a 39-year-old Bangladeshi Work Permit holder, who showed first symptoms of COVID-19 one week before his diagnosis on 8 February (Sim and Kok, 2020). Although the construction worker had, while he was infectious, visited Mustafa Centre, a bustling 24-hour food and retail shopping centre located in Little India, no immediate spike in symptomatic cases was recorded in relation to Case 42 (Phua, 2020b).

Only in hindsight did public health authorities view Mustafa Centre as a potential site of mass infection, contributing to the evident rise in COVID-19 cases in late March. By early April, imported cases and so-called community cases (occurring outside the dormitories) had remained constant in a low double-digit range. Virus control and the comparatively low number of new infections were largely ascribed to the government's strategy of "mitigation and containment", notably isolating cases and meticulously tracing clusters and new infections.

Civil society activist groups, such as TWC2, had repeatedly and very publicly raised concern about the serious challenges of applying a "mitigation and containment" strategy if there were to be a pandemic outbreak in the dormitories, where cramped living conditions made social distancing virtually impossible. On 23 March 2020, TWC2 published an open letter in *The Straits Times*, warning of the fatal consequences of COVID-19 spreading in the dorms (TWC2, 2020a). As public health academic Alex

Cook shared in an interview with Channel News Asia (Phua, 2020b): "There were few voices who sounded the alarm, and I will admit to not having the dorms on my radar at the start of the outbreak". COVID-19 cases quadrupled in the first two weeks of April 2020. From just 10 migrant workers out of all 1,000 cases on 1 April, the share of migrant workers' COVID-19 infections rose to 60% of the total 4,427 cases recorded on 16 April (MOH, 2020). The government recognized the urgency and responded to the rapid increase in COVID-19 cases by issuing a first two-week lockdown and isolation notice to two of the most affected dormitories, S11@Pungol and Westlite Toh Guan from 5 April (Sen and Ong, 2020). The announcement of a "three-pronged strategy" on 14 April (MOH, 2020) led to a full lockdown for all purpose-built dormitories, while isolating positive cases and shifting healthy and essential workers to alternative accommodation, including military camps, empty housing blocks, and other facilities (Koh, 2020).

Meanwhile, MOM sent out so-called Forward Assurance and Support Teams (FAST). Comprising personnel from the Singapore Armed Forces, the Police Force, and MOM, they assisted dorm operators with resident management during the lockdown, including food distribution, medical service provision, and support with employment-related issues, such as salary payments (Singapore Government, 2020b). The government was also able to quickly mobilize NGOs for assistance (Poh, 2020). Due to the high rate of infections and their vast size, purpose-built dormitories quickly became the hotspots of emergency response. From anecdotal evidence provided by frontline personnel, the situation in the different dormitories varied drastically.

Language barriers and communication gaps between migrant workers, dorm operators, and government authorities not only led to a delay in the relay of messages, but in many instances to crucially missing information on migrant workers' whereabouts in the midst of their constant moving between various dorm sites, as employers told various news outlets (Phua, 2020b). Recalling his experience at the frontline, Dr Jeremy Lim, vice-chairman of HealthServe, a non-governmental organization looking after the needs of migrant workers, pointed to a lack of sufficient manpower and the fear of migrant worker unrest due to dissatisfaction about the shortage and quality of their distributed meals early on during the lockdown (Lim, 2020). Nonetheless, despite the miscommunication and numerous challenges in the daily micromanagement of dormitories under lockdown, different stakeholders commended the efforts undertaken by both public and private actors to maintain a problem-solving attitude and cooperation over the first learning-phase of lockdown (Cai, Y. 2020).

With strict lockdown measures and the provision of mass testing, the government was able by 1 June 2020 to declare 60 dormitories, housing a total of 8,000 residents, "cleared" of COVID-19, while an additional 32,000 workers hosted at alternative lodging sites were allowed to resume work. Although increasing numbers of foreign workers returned to their workplaces, their movement remained significantly restricted. Within many dormitories, the facilitation of social distancing was driven by new technology adaptations, such as the obligatory scanning of QR codes at doors of different floor levels to both improve traceability of potentially asymptomatic patients and simultaneously prevent overcrowding in specific areas. Such close monitoring of entries and exits and the tracking of workers' circulation has thereby led to an increased surveillance of migrant workers' movements.

Beyond the dormitories, migrant workers remained subjected to an "employer consent rule". The regulation, which received criticism by migrant worker activist groups HOME and TWC2 (2020d) and was subsequently revised on 3 August 2020, required employers to "not allow, or cause to be allowed, the foreign employee … to leave the dormitory unless the employer is satisfied that the foreign employee — (a) has permission from the Controller to do so; or (b) is seeking medical treatment" (MOM, 2020f). Migrant workers voiced their discontent about the infringement of their right to movement and access to basic services, reporting it to different NGOs operating on the ground (TWC2, 2020d).

Although many dormitories had been "cleared" of COVID-19 by late July, a spike in new cases in early August led to new lockdowns for several dormitories from 12 August. In order to cope with future outbreaks and increased contamination, the government moved to build more dormitories more quickly in order to distribute migrant workers to more spacious accommodation with improved living standards. In the meantime, migrant workers were at the mercy of their employers, who decided on their rest days at designated recreational centres (TWC2, 2020g). While the Singaporean public at large moved steadily towards "Phase 3" following a two-month partial lockdown, also known as the "circuit breaker", many migrant workers continued in effect to be in a prolonged lockdown with great uncertainty as to when they would return to a new normal.

UNCERTAINTY AND MENTAL DISTRESS

Migrant workers have been depicted predominantly in a third-person narrative throughout the pandemic, in many ways objectified, stripped of their agency, and left with numerous COVID-19-related concerns about their job security, salary pay-out, and subsistence (Chok, n.d.).

According to activists, migrant workers had not viewed the dormitory layout and its allocation of cramped living space as a major issue prior to the COVID-19 outbreak. Yet, the long confinement under the described living conditions has had a significant impact on the workers' mental and physical well-being. Cai Yinzhou (2020), representative of the COVID-19 Migrant Support Coalition, explained how, during the early stages of lockdown, uncertainty about the pandemic situation and their employment left them very troubled. This was exacerbated by a delay in the translation of official communication. Although NGOs, public healthcare staff, and FAST personnel were quickly mobilized to provide emergency support in the dormitories, ground personnel remained critically short-staffed. Jolovan Wham (2020), in his role as social worker for HOME, described the situation as "firefighting" on all fronts. TWC2 vice-president Alex Au (2020) highlighted the "complete collapse of MOM" in terms of lack of staff and unpreparedness to deal with a pandemic outbreak in the dormitories.

Jeremy Lim (2020), whose organization HealthServe was at the dormitories to provide emergency relief, noted a high risk of riots in the early stages of lockdown, when migrant workers complained about food quality and malfunctioning distribution schemes. TWC2 president Debbie Fordyce (2020) described how the strict regulations on food packaging and closure of all communal kitchens created a large accumulation of plastic waste in dormitory rooms.

On the one hand, migrant worker accounts, as transmitted by activist groups and ground staff, demonstrated comprehension and acceptance of government measures and the strict, prolonged lockdown for a "greater good" (Jeremy Lim, personal communication, 2020). On the other hand, migrant workers have experienced heightened mental distress throughout the lockdown period. Such mental anguish, for many an even greater threat than the virus itself (TWC2, 2020f), must be linked to both the immediate uncertainty experienced during the pandemic, including concerns over salary payment, remittances, and debts, as much as a deeper, structural precarity that is the product of a neoliberal low-waged migrant management.

Suicides and suicidal intents were captured in a number of videos and pictures of migrant workers standing close to bridge railings and rooftop ledges, as well as photos of migrant workers engaging in self-harm (Business Times, 2020). From April to August 2020, seven suspected suicides including attempts were registered. Yet, in responding to the events and public concerns, MOM stated that it did not "observe a spike in the number of migrant worker suicides compared to the previous year" (Cai, L., 2020). In November 2020, the new government task force "Project Dawn" (MOM, 2020d) was announced to address and raise awareness of depression among migrant workers. It remains to be seen whether the project manages to overcome existing cultural and language barriers and provide the much-needed mental health support.

In the meantime, a number of migrant workers openly voiced their anguish and staged protest against the post-circuit-breaker mandatory "employer consent" for moving beyond the confines of the dormitories. Comparing their situation with slave-like conditions, they changed their profile pictures on social media (Cai, Y., 2020). With limited agency, such small acts of resistance reflected the workers' conflicted standing vis-à-vis both COVID-19 as exogenous shock and its endogenous repercussions on individual rights and obligations within the contract labour management system. At the same time, migrant workers have increasingly resorted to apps such as TikTok to share glimpses of daily life in the dormitories under lockdown and to provide and receive mutual support to and from other workers around the world (Chua, 2020).

Civic Activism for the Migrant Worker Cause

Given migrant workers' limited agency and general fear of speaking up, NGOs have for decades played a significant role in improving their well-being. When COVID-19 struck, this extended to the provision of immediate relief and emergency response, as well as facilitating access to public healthcare and legal services.

There are at least four key organizations related to the migrant worker cause: Humanitarian Organization for Migration Economics (HOME), Transient Workers Count Too (TWC2), Migrant Workers' Centre (MWC), and HealthServe. At one end of the spectrum, HOME and TWC2 have been vocal about the systemic nature of migrant worker precarity and the government's failure to bring about structural change (TWC2, 2020e). At the other end, MWC is a quasi-government organization funded by the National Trade Union Congress (Singapore's only trade union centre and one that is closely aligned to the ruling People's Action Party [PAP]) and is thus much less independent of the state. Meanwhile, HealthServe has taken a less ideological approach, focusing purely on health-related concerns (Lim, 2020).

According to Wham (2020), the government employed a "divide and rule" strategy by granting only those NGOs that were less advocacy-oriented access to the dormitories at the height of the infections. This was done even though non-governmental support and manpower were critically needed to provide immediate relief, engage in research-based advocacy, and run public awareness-raising campaigns. Although they were "struggling under the weight of the problem", NGOs—according to Wham (2020)—did not cease to assist in whatever ways that they could. Along with the ad-hoc COVID-19 Migrant Support Coalition (CMSC), NGOs provided services such as tele-counselling and supported workers facing contract or salary issues. Given the high number of cases of workers not being paid their salaries, especially in the post-lockdown period, there was increased demand for case work and legal counselling services (TWC2, 2020f). HOME and TWC2 have continuously been advocating for an improved dormitory design that should provide more privacy notwithstanding limited allocation of room size per worker, citing such best practices from dormitory set-ups in Japan where cross mixing and infection transmissions could be contained (Au, 2020).

Beyond the question of dormitory re-design and reform, NGO representatives have been concerned about an intensification of spatial segregation through the construction of new dormitories. TWC2 president Debbie Fordyce noted the implications on basic freedom and mental well-being of new surveillance mechanisms as part of COVID-19 tracing strategies (Fordyce, 2020).

Overall, migrant worker organizations have played an essential role in standing up for migrant workers' concerns, revealing underlying tensions in Singapore's labour migration management. They have raised public awareness and, in some instances, achieved modest policy change, including the ongoing discussions on improving dormitory living standards (Phua, 2020a). Their efforts are met by a range of public perceptions and attitudes, from appreciative support to blatant moral panic, mirrored in media discourse.

Public Perception and Media Discourse

Media reporting as well as the daily official updates on COVID-19 cases have reflected and reinforced an "us vs. them" mentality. Each day, Singaporeans have been receiving news of infections where the rates are separated clearly between non-imported community cases and dormitory residents cases. Reflecting spatial segregation between Singapore's society and migrant workers, such a form of reporting reinforced social boundaries between a perceived Singaporean "community" and the migrant worker "out-group".

In the context of the pandemic, both subtle and blatant criticism of migrant workers and dormitory conditions could be observed across different media platforms, nourishing their portrayal as the "heterotopian other". An opinion piece on 13 April 2020 in the Chinese daily *Lianhe Zaobao*, the country's largest Chinese newspaper, caused a backlash from more progressive Singaporeans. While lauding the government's efforts to curb the spread of the virus, the author of the commentary urged migrant workers to exercise personal responsibility:

> The crux is, did the workers in these dormitories do their part? Is their personal hygiene up to standard? Did they clear up after themselves after they used the kitchen? Did they keep the toilet clean after using it? [...]] If personal hygiene efforts don't improve, things will remain the same wherever they go. (Lianhe Zaobao, 2020, translated by Yong Han Poh)

In framing the pandemic spread mainly as a matter of personal hygiene and employing illustrations of the "dirty foreigner" as part of a "them-group", the author focused the question of responsibility on to the migrant workers themselves. Even Law and Home Affairs Minister K. Shanmugam criticized the letter as revealing "underlying racism" (Mahmud, 2020).

Similarly, on social media platforms, moral panic rhetoric and polarized opinions surrounding the outbreak in the dormitories were tied to the same kinds of stereotypes and stigmas that are observed in the narrative of the Little India riots. In public profiles and groups on Facebook, it was not difficult to find references to a lack of basic self-hygiene, "a thing, which they really need to learn" (J.C., 2020), or to a culture or habit of living together "in a place crawling with ants and cockroaches" (J.T., 2020). Some posts, such as the following, were accusatory:

now because government looking into dormitory's hygiene due to COVID-19, these workers become very upset about their current living conditions. They jump on the opportunity to gain something out of it. (J.T., 2020)

At the other end of the spectrum, several community initiatives were mobilized, exemplifying positive attitudes and support for migrant workers, especially during the circuit breaker. In April 2020, SGforForeignWorkers started collecting and translating notes written by Singaporeans directed to migrant workers. The bottom-up initiative aimed to provide a platform to "build a stronger, collective Singaporean voice valuing migrant workers" (Ng, 2020). Project Belanja and Maskforce organized food deliveries and masks to migrant workers' accommodations (including dormitories), thanks to private donations (Toh, 2020). As of November 2020, Maskforce raised $62,258 from 234 donors and Belanja sponsored over 7,000 meals from April to August 2020 (GivingSg, 2020).

The general appreciation of migrant workers and their role in Singapore's economic development contrasts with the approach of isolating them in dedicated spaces instead of aiming for greater integration into Singapore society. However, narratives of migrant workers as threats in the media underline the populist value of security in terms of protection against the perceived risk coming from "outside". The perceived threats and populist fears have not led to significant restrictions on the number of migrant workers allowed to enter Singapore, due to a pragmatic rationale undergirding the country's reliance on them. However, they translate into spatial separation between the Singaporean community and migrant workers in dormitories located in Singapore's periphery.

The Government as Pragmatic Mediator

Amidst NIMBY campaigns on the one hand and pressure from pro-migrant-worker NGOs on the other hand, the government has tried pragmatically to mediate between moral panic and inclusive community activism. Its pragmatic approach is especially evident in moving migrant workers to residential accommodations in the wake of the pandemic until new dormitories could be constructed. In spite of public resistance to such efforts to integrate migrant workers into residential neighbourhoods, no matter how temporary the arrangement, the government moved ahead with its decision while keeping space optimization as the guiding principle in land-scarce Singapore, arguing that "it is inevitable that some of the new dorm sites will be … near residential areas" ("Coronavirus: Singapore must reject", 2020). Minister Lawrence Wong, then co-chair of the multi-ministry task force on COVID-19, conveyed Singapore's appreciation of "the contribution that our migrant workers have made, and will continue to make, in building Singapore". He urged Singaporeans to "welcome them as part of our community" and to "do our part to reject the 'not in my backyard mindset'". The government has continuously called for greater tolerance and backed the social media campaign #WelcomeInMy-Backyard, initiated by a group of Singaporeans, whose platform invites Singaporeans to post notes of appreciation and welcome directed at migrant workers ("Coronavirus: Singapore must reject", 2020).

Official government rhetoric mirrors the public appreciation of migrant workers from within a segment of Singapore society. However, the mere recognition of their contribution to the economy's growth does not translate in practice to deeper structural reform, whether of foreign labour policies or even migrant dormitory regulations. The gap between public discourse and policy realities on the ground reflects the government's pragmatic approach, weighing perceived risks and cost against potential benefits, either in monetary terms or electoral gains, to best manage migrant workers' employment and life in Singapore.

Given the scarcity of space, the high reliance on low-waged migrant workers, and the current precarious housing situation that facilitates the spread of the virus, the government has taken the role of a paternalistic mediator in partially addressing opposing demands. First, public pressure and moral panic are addressed through the promise of the future construction of fully integrated dormitories in the periphery, which will provide a suite of amenities and services, such as recreation centres, hairdressers, and shops, basically to eliminate the need for migrant workers to venture outside of the dormitories. This will exacerbate spatial segregation. Second, while NGO demands for improved housing are unlikely to be implemented via the granting of more legal rights, the government is likely to build new flagship dormitories with improved standards.

Dormitories of the Future

A number of architects and scholars have been strong advocates of improved living standards in migrant worker dormitories. Imran Bin Tajudeen highlighted a double standard when it came to approaching migrant worker dormitories on the one hand, and barracks built for the

Singapore Armed Forces on the other, at least where ventilation and natural lightning were concerned. The latter were "much more provisioned in terms of the living space standards" (Aldgra, 2020). Veteran architect Tay Kheng Soon argued that foreign worker dormitories "have to be healthy places [...], similar to [National Service] dorms which have proven unproblematic given adequate toilets and showers, cross ventilation and proper upkeep" (Del Rosario, 2020). Tay equated migrant workers with soldiers performing compulsory military service (or National Service) in terms of their contribution to Singapore's development: "army dorms and FW dorms should be similarly considered as part of the national infrastructure and funded accordingly". Tay also recommended that the state acquire all dormitories, upgrade them to increase resilience and preparedness for future pandemics, replace degenerated dormitories, and construct new ones (Del Rosario, 2020).

Among the more radical ideas was one to build so-called floating dormitories. Platforms of reinforced concrete that can be connected to one another would address Singapore's space scarcity, lighten the stress and strain on urban infrastructure, and overcome the problem of overcrowding in conventional dormitories, providing each resident "8 to 9 m^2 of exclusive space" (Heng, 2020a). Two floating accommodations in Tanjong Pagar Terminal, that had been used in offshore and marine work, were already being used during the pandemic to house non-infected workers (MPA, 2020). Singapore's Society of Floating Solutions highlighted the benefit of floating clusters that can be manoeuvred close to work sites, further saving costs while preventing interaction with Singapore's "mainland residents". Floating dormitories are innovative and lucrative businesses that could be connected to commercial floating platforms, on which recreational parks including food outlets, barbecue pits, and jogging facilities could be built (Heng, 2020b). Such solutions appear as a well-suited win–win solution for the Singaporean migration management narrative, not only in terms of future pandemic preparedness, but also with regard to space maximization and spatial segregation.

Conclusion

The COVID-19 spread in migrant worker dormitories offers a new lens to observe and reveal the multifaceted structures and practices of migrant worker management grounded in a neoliberal and pragmatic approach in Singapore. Pragmatism and capitalist market practices translate into a highly efficient use and optimisation of the city's scarce space. Long before the pandemic outbreak, migrant worker dormitories in Singapore were a heterotopia of spatial and social segregation. Against this conceptual background, the dormitories' embodiment of the precarity of place has led to numerous underlying societal tensions, which have been picked up by public rhetoric during the pandemic.

In the early days of the pandemic outbreak, Singapore was praised for its quick and presumably efficient response. However, with the spikes of cases in foreign worker dormitories in early to mid-April 2020, the initial positive image experienced backlash. International media reports on the high rates of infections in dormitories highlighted the government's loss of control while in many ways forgetting that "migrant workers are people" (Han, 2020; "Infections deluge", 2020; Leung, 2020). Hence, these dormitories have emerged as spaces of opposing perceptions and reactions, notably moral panic and community support. While populist discourse has fuelled the perceived "foreign threat", local initiatives have continuously upheld recognition and appreciation of migrant workers while providing direct support.

In this realm of contestation, the Singaporean government performs pragmatic mediation. On the one hand, NGO and public concerns are appeased with official rhetoric. On the other hand, NIMBY mentality and xenophobic attitudes are condemned. However, beyond public discourse and rhetoric, no systemic policy change has been initiated to address migrant workers' underlying precarities that have existed for decades, the result of attachment to neoliberal globalization. On the contrary, the more cost-efficient approach to treating symptoms in the short term without tackling root concerns in the long term only underpins the critical observation of COVID-19 as a pandemic of inequality in Singapore.

REFERENCES

Aldgra, F. (2020) Why the double standard between how army barracks and migrant worker dormitories are built, asks Dr Imran Tajudeen. *The Online Citizen Asia*, 6 May. https://toca.wpengine.com/2020/05/06/why-the-double-standard-between-how-army-barracks-and-migrant-worker-dormit ories-are-built-asks-dr-imran-tajudeen/. Accessed 19 November 2020.

Allport, G. W. (1954) *The nature of prejudice.* Cambridge/Reading, MA: Addison-Wesley.

Anderson, B. (1983) *Imagined communities: Reflections on the origin and spread of nationalism*. New York: Verso.

Ang, J. et al. (2019) Are migrant workers in Singapore receiving adequate healthcare? A survey of doctors working in public tertiary healthcare institutions. *Singapore Medical Journal*, 61(10), 540–547. https://doi.org/10.11622/smedj.2019101.

Baey, G., and Yeoh, B. S. A. (2015) *Migration and precarious work: Negotiating debt, employment, and livelihood strategies amongst Bangladeshi migrant men working in Singapore's construction industry*. Migrating Out of Poverty Working Paper 26. http://www.migratingoutofpoverty.org/files/file.php?name=wp26-baey-yeoh-2015-migration-and-precarious-work.pdf&site=354. Accessed 13 October 2020.

Baey, G., and Yeoh, B. S. A. (2018) "The lottery of my life": Migration trajectories and the production of precarity among Bangladeshi migrant workers in Singapore's construction industry. *Asian and Pacific Migration Journal*, 27(3), 249–272. https://doi.org/10.1177/0117196818780087.

Bal, C. (2017) Myths and facts: Migrant workers in Singapore. *New Naratif*, 9 September. https://newnaratif.com/research/myths-and-facts-migrant-workers-in-singapore/#_ftn49. Accessed 20 October 2020.

Banki, S. (2013) Precarity of place: A complement to the growing precariat literature. *Global Discourse*, 3(3–4), 450–463. https://doi.org/10.1080/23269995.2014.881139.

Cai, L. (2020) MOH: Tackling mental health and anxiety of migrant workers is an on-going process. *Online Citizen Asia*, 7 August. https://www.onlinecitizenasia.com/2020/08/07/lawrence-wong-tackling-mental-health-and-anxiety-of-migrant-workers-is-an-on-going-process/. Accessed 18 October 2020.

Chin, C. (2019) Precarious work and its complicit network: Migrant labour in Singapore. *Journal of Contemporary Asia*, 49(4), 528–551. https://doi.org/10.1080/00472336.2019.1572209.

Chin, C., Chow, C., and Tay, T. (2020) The next generation foreign workers' dormitory. *Edge Prop*, 8 May. https://www.edgeprop.sg/property-news/next-generation-foreign-workers%E2%80%99-dormitory. Accessed 17 November 2020.

Chok, S. (2017) *Wage theft & exploitation among Singapore's migrant workers*. Home Position Paper, January 2017. https://static1.squarespace.com/static/5a12725612abd96b9c737354/t/5a1fce6f652dead776d3c970/1512033911372/Position_Paper_Wage-Theft-Exploitation-among-Singapores-Migrant-Workers.pdf. Accessed 19 October 2020.

Chok, S. (n.d.) Policy brief: Protecting migrant workers' rights in the midst of Covid-19. *HOME*. https://www.home.org.sg/statements/2020/4/15/policy-brief-protecting-migrant-workers-rights-in-the-midst-of-covid-19. Accessed 18 October 2020.

Chua, E. (2020) Staying plugged in: Video app TikTok gives migrant workers a means to stay connected for support. *The Straits Times*, 26 October. https://www.straitstimes.com/singapore/staying-plugged-in-video-app-tiktok-gives-migrant-workers-a-means-to-stay-connected-for.

CMSC. (2020) *COVID-19 Migrant support coalition.* https://www.sgmigrant.com/en-covid19. Accessed 20 October 2020.

Coronavirus: Singapore must reject "not in my backyard" mindset when rehousing migrant workers, top official says. (2020) *South China Morning Post*, 11 June. https://www.scmp.com/news/asia/southeast-asia/article/308 8486/coronavirus-singapore-must-reject-not-my-backyard-mindset. Accessed 25 October 2020.

Del Rosario, B. (2020) Veteran architect: Foreign worker dorms should be similar to NS dorms. *The Independent*, 18 April. https://theindependent.sg/veteran-architect-foreign-worker-dorms-should-be-similar-to-ns-dorms/. Accessed 17 November 2020.

Dutta, M. J., Tan, N., and Kaur, S. (2016) Media, migration and politics: The coverage of the Little India Riot in The Straits Times in Singapore. *Journal of Creative Communications*, 11(1), 26–43. https://doi.org/10.1177/097325 8616630214.

Foucault, M. (1984) Des espaces autres. *Architecture, Mouvement, Continuité*, 5, 46–49 (1984).

GivingSG. (2020) Maskforce. https://www.giving.sg/campaigns/maskforce. Accessed 18 November 2020.

Goh, Daniel P. S. (2014) The Little India Riot and the spatiality of migrant labor in Singapore. *Society and Space Magazine*, 8 September. https://www.societyandspace.org/articles/the-little-india-riot-and-the-spatiality-of-migrant-labor-in-singapore. Accessed 16 October 2020.

Goode, E., and Ben-Yahuda, N. (2009) *Moral panics: The social construction of deviance* (2nd ed.). Oxford: Wiley-Blackwell.

Han, K. (2020) Singapore is trying to forget migrant workers are people. *Foreign Policy*, 6 May. https://foreignpolicy.com/2020/05/06/singapore-coronavirus-pandemic-migrant-workers/. Accessed 17 November 2020.

Hamid, W., and Tutt, D. (2019) "Thrown away like a banana leaf": Precarity of labour and precarity of place for Tamil migrant construction workers in Singapore. *Construction Management and Economics*, 37(9), 513–536. https://doi.org/10.1080/01446193.2019.1595075.

Hamidi, S., Sabouri, S., and Reid, E. (2020) Does density aggravate the Covid-19 pandemic? *Journal of the American Planning Association*, 86 (4), 495–509. https://doi.org/10.1080/01944363.2020.1777891.

Heng, L. S. (2020a) A floating dorm for workers: An idea that merits consideration. *The Straits Time*, 23 May. https://www.straitstimes.com/opinion/a-floating-dorm-for-workers-an-idea-that-merits-consideration. Accessed 17 November 2020.

Heng, L. S. (2020b) Post Covid 19 housing for migrant workers, Addressing their psychological and physical needs. President's Message, 35/2020. *Society of Floating Solutions, Singapore*. https://floatingsolutions.org/presidents-message/. Accessed 18 November 2020.

Infections deluge at Singapore housing for foreign workers. (2020) *The Standard*, 17 April. https://www.thestandard.com.hk/section-news/section/11/218240/Infection-deluge-at-Singapore-housing-for-foreign-workers. Accessed 18 November 2020.

International Labor Organization (ILO). (2019). Public attitudes towards migrant workers in Japan, Malaysia, Singapore, and Thailand. https://www.ilo.org/wcmsp5/groups/public/---asia/---ro-bangkok/documents/publication/wcms_732443.pdf. Accessed 30 September 2020.

J.C. (2020) S11 Dormitory condition please take a look how is our Singapore standard of Domitory condition, comment on Facebook Post, shared on 06 April. https://www.facebook.com/jason.see.56/posts/10156104889297395. Accessed 20 November 2020.

J.T. (2020) S11 Dormitory condition please take a look how is our Singapore standard of Domitory condition, Comment on Facebook Post, shared on 06 April. https://www.facebook.com/jason.see.56/posts/10156104889297395. Accessed 20 November, 2020.

Koh, D. (2020) Migrant workers and COVID-19. *Occupational and Environ Medicine*, 77(9), 634–636. https://doi.org/10.1136/oemed-2020-106626.

Lafazani, O. (2013) A border within a border: The migrant's squatter settlement in Patras as a heterotopia. *Journal of Borderlands Studies*, 28(1), 1–13. https://doi.org/10.1080/08865655.2012.751731.

Lee, W. et al. (2014) Health-seeking behaviour of male foreign migrant workers living in a dormitory in Singapore. *BMC Health Services Research*, 14, 300. https://doi.org/10.1186/1472-6963-14-300.

Lefebvre, H. (2009) (ed. Brenner, N. and Elden, S) *State, space, world: Selected essays*. University of Minnesota Press, Minneapolis.

Leung, H. (2020) Why Singapore, once a model for Coronavirus response, lost control of its outbreak. *Time*, 20 April. https://time.com/5824039/singapore-outbreak-migrant-workers/. Accessed 17 November 2020.

Ling, S. (2020) TWC2: Condition of the migrant worker's dormitories nearly ideal for transmission of infection. *The Online Citizen Asia*, 7 April. https://www.onlinecitizenasia.com/2020/04/07/twc2-condition-of-the-migrant-workers-dormitories-nearly-ideal-for-transmission-of-infection/. Accessed 14 October 2020.

Loong, S. (2020) Who is responsible for Singapore's migrant workers, and why does it matter? *Academia SG*, 5 May. https://www.academia.sg/academic-views/who-is-responsible-for-singapores-migrant-workers-and-why-does-it-matter/. Accessed 18 November 2020.

Mahmud, A. H. (2020) COVID-19: Forum letter on foreign worker dormitory cases reveals 'underlying racism', says Shanmugam. *Channel News Asia*, 18 April. https://www.channelnewsasia.com/news/singapore/covid-19-letter-zaobao-foreign-worker-dormitory-racism-shanmugam-12654924. Accessed 20 November 2020.

Maritime and Port Authority of Singapore (MPA). (2020) Singapore to add floating accommodation to range of housing for foreign workers. https://www.mpa.gov.sg/web/portal/home/media-centre/news-releases/detail/6c4510c3-0527-4dc6-b687-cc8dfc0ad001. Accessed 16 November 2020.

Ministry of Health (MOH). (2020) Updates on COVID-19 (Coronavirus Disease 2019) local situation. https://www.moh.gov.sg/covid-19. Accessed 2 November 2020.

Ministry of Manpower (MOM). (2020a) Ministerial statement by Mrs Josephine Teo, Minister for Manpower, 4 May 2020. https://www.mom.gov.sg/newsroom/parliament-questions-and-replies/2020/0504-ministerial-statement-by-mrs-josephine-teo-minister-for-manpower-4-may-2020. Accessed 5 November 2020.

Ministry of Manpower (MOM). (2020b) Foreign workforce numbers. https://www.mom.gov.sg/documents-and-publications/foreign-workforce-numbers. Accessed 27 September 2020.

Ministry of Manpower (MOM). (2020c) Various types of housing and their specific requirements. https://www.mom.gov.sg/passes-and-permits/work-permit-for-foreign-worker/housing/various-types-of-housing. Accessed 6 October 2020.

Ministry of Manpower (MOM). (2020d) New taskforce to enhance mental health care support for migrant workers. https://www.mom.gov.sg/newsroom/press-releases/2020/1106-new-taskforce-to-enhance-mental-health-care-support-for-migrant-workers.

Ministry of Manpower (MOM). (2020e) List of foreign worker dormitories. Available at: https://www.mom.gov.sg/passes-and-permits/work-permit-for-foreign-worker/housing/foreign-worker-dormitories#/?page=1&q. Accessed 14 November 2020.

Ministry of Manpower (MOM). (2020f) Employment of foreign manpower (Work passes) regulations 2012. status [S 427/2020 wef 02/06/2020]. https://sso.agc.gov.sg/SL/EFMA1990-S569-2012?DocDate=20200601#Sc4-. Accessed 29 June 2020.

Neilson, B., and Rossiter, N. (2006) From precarity to precariousness and back again: Labour, life and unstable networks. *Variant*, 25(2), 10–13.

Ng, N. M. (2020) How you can pledge to help migrant workers in Singapore right now. *TimeOut*, 3 June. https://www.timeout.com/singapore/things-to-do/how-to-help-migrant-workers-in-singapore?awc=16830_160340 0987_c94c3d47ac138c74cb25ce42a7ab0115. Accessed 21 October 2020.

Phua, R. (2020a) COVID-19: Singapore to build new dormitories with improved living standards for migrant workers. *Channel News Asia*, 1 June. https://www.channelnewsasia.com/news/singapore/covid-19-sin gapore-new-dormitories-foreign-workers-conditions-12792538. Accessed 18 November 2020.

Phua, R. (2020b) In focus: The long, challenging journey to bring COVID-19 under control in migrant worker dormitories. *Channel News Asia*, 11 September. https://www.channelnewsasia.com/news/singapore/in-focus-cov id19-singapore-migrant-worker-dormitories-lockdown-13081210. Accessed 24 October 2020.

Poh, Y. H. (2020) Singapore's migrant worker debate: Advocacy amid a pandemic. *The Diplomat*, 12 April. https://thediplomat.com/2020/04/singapores-migrant-worker-debate-advocacy-amid-a-pandemic/. Accessed 24 October 2020.

Ratcliffe, R. (2020) Singapore's cramped migrant worker dorms hide Covid-19 surge risk. *The Guardian*, 17 April. https://www.theguardian.com/world/2020/apr/17/singapores-cramped-migrant-worker-dorms-hide-covid-19-surge-risk. Accessed 19 October 2020.

Sadarangani, S., Poh, L. L., and Vasoo, S. (2017) Infectious diseases and migrant worker health in Singapore: A receiving country's perspective. *Journal of Travel Medicine*, 1–9.

Sen, N. J., and Ong, J. (2020) The big read: Solving Singapore's foreign workers problem requires serious soul searching, from top to bottom. *Channel News Asia*, 11 May. https://www.channelnewsasia.com/news/singapore/cor onavirus-covid-19-foreign-workers-big-read-dormitories-12718880. Accessed 5 October 2020.

Sibley, D. (1995) *Geographies of exclusion: Society and difference in the West*. London: New York.

Sim, C. (2015) Little India Riot. *Singapore Infopedia*. https://www.resear chgate.net/publication/26490721_From_Precarity_to_Precariousness_and_Back_Again_Labour_Life_and_Unstable_Networks. Accessed 17 November 2020.

Sim, D., and Kok, X. (2020) How did migrant worker dorms become Singapore's biggest Covid-19 cluster? *South China Morning Post*, 17 April. https://www.scmp.com/week-asia/explained/article/3080466/how-did-migrant-worker-dormitories-become-singapores-biggest. Accessed 7 October 2020.

Singapore Migrant Worker Mental Health in Spotlight after Self Harm Incident. (2020) *Business Times*, 5 August. https://www.businesstimes.com.sg/govern ment-economy/singapore-migrant-worker-mental-health-in-spotlight-after-self-harm-incident. Accessed 5 October 2020.

Singapore Government. (2020a) Total persons, locals and foreigners arrested: Persons arrested by group. https://data.gov.sg/dataset/total-persons-loc als-and-foreigners-arrested?resource_id=bdd267bf-2ded-4ed7-8834-08b4ec 977e7a. Accessed 17 November 2020.

Singapore Government. (2020b, May 19) Pulling together fast to ensure the well-being of migrant workers. MCI—Gov.SG. https://www.gov.sg/article/ pulling-together-fast-to-ensure-the-well-being-of-migrant-workers. Accessed 18 October 2020.

Tan, Y. (2020) Covid-19 Singapore: A 'pandemic of inequality' exposed. *BBC News*, 17 September. https://www.bbc.com/news/world-asia-54082861. Accessed 3 October 2020.

The Straits Time. (1983) Jayakumar tells why foreign workers must go. *The Straits Times*, 7 November.

Toh, W. L. (2020) Coronavirus: Local firms step up to help foreign workers amid pandemic. *The Straits Time*, 25 April. https://www.straitstimes.com/ singapore/coronavirus-local-firms-step-up-to-help-foreign-workers-amid-pan demic. Accessed 24 October 2020.

TWC2. (2020a) Straits times forum: Employers' practices leave foreign workers vulnerable to infection, 23 March. https://twc2.org.sg/2020/03/23/str aits-times-forum-employers-practices-leave-foreign-workers-vulnerable-to-inf ection/. Accessed 27 September 2020.

TWC2. (2020b) Covid-19: Media statement, 13 April. https://twc2.org. sg/2020/04/13/covid-19-media-statement-13-april-2020-longer-version/. Accessed 27 September 2020.

TWC2. (2020c) How many employers are there?, 4 May. https://twc2.org.sg/ 2020/05/04/how-many-employers-are-there/. Accessed 4 October 2020.

TWC2. (2020d) Post-Covid law makes migrant workers prisoners of employers, 29 June. https://twc2.org.sg/2020/06/29/post-covid-law-makes-migrant-workers-prisoners-of-employers/. Accessed 4 October 2020.

TWC2. (2020e) Migrant bodies sacrificed on the altar of self-praise, 3 August. https://twc2.org.sg/2020/08/03/migrant-bodies-sacrificed-on-the-altar-of-self-praise/. Accessed 10 October 2020.

TWC2. (2020f) Five questions from reporters, 5 August. https://twc2.org.sg/ 2020/08/05/five-questions-from-reporters/. Accessed 9 October 2020.

TWC2. (2020g) Research finding: Only a handful of workers have had rest days out from dorms, 17 September. https://twc2.org.sg/2020/09/17/ research-finding-only-a-handful-of-workers-have-had-rest-days-out-from-dorms/. Accessed 10 October 2020.

Wee, K., Goh, C., and Yeoh, B. S. A. (2018) Chutes-and-ladders: The migration industry, conditionality, and the production of precarity among migrant domestic workers in Singapore. *Journal of Ethnic and Migration Studies*, 45(14), 2672–2688. https://doi.org/10.1080/1369183x.2018.1528099.
Zieleniec, A. (2007) *Space and social theory*. Los Angeles: Sage.

Interviews

Au, Alex (2020) Personal communication, 14 October [Interview].
Cai, Yinzhou (2020) Personal communication, 29 September [Interview].
Fordyce, Debbie (2020) Personal communication, 13 October [Interview].
Lim, Jeremy (2020) Personal communication, 13 October [Interview].
Wham, Jolovan (2020) Personal communication, 20 September [Interview].

CHAPTER 7

Ready for the Post-Pandemic World?

Kenneth Paul Tan

Abstract The migrant worker dormitory clusters, although certainly a serious matter, might seem like just a blemish in an otherwise stellar record of successful crisis management by a high-capacity government responsible for developing Singapore from a "Third World" to a "First World" country in a very short period. Made up of very capable technocrats with a pragmatic outlook, this government focused on results, were quick to react to problems as they surfaced, and never took its eye away from the unsentimental task of keeping its globally embedded economy going as a vital part of national survival. Some might argue, further, that the authorities and countless other people in Singapore who volunteered their support did the best they could, in the context of an unprecedented and unpredictable pandemic of this scale and magnitude. However, the dormitory clusters and other lapses are symptoms of deeper structural problems. This is an important perspective that can constructively provide insight into whether these kinds of problems will

K. P. Tan (✉)
School of Communication and Film, Hong Kong Baptist University, Kowloon Tong, Hong Kong
e-mail: kennethptan@hkbu.edu.hk

© The Author(s), under exclusive license to Springer Nature Singapore Pte Ltd. 2022
K. P. Tan (ed.), *Singapore's First Year of COVID-19*,
https://doi.org/10.1007/978-981-19-0368-7_7

manifest again and again in occasional eruptions and disruptions, which are painful but manageable. Or whether they will lead to more systemically destructive outcomes over time, which will either ruin Singapore eventually or create the opportunity to rebuild something better. Given Singapore's track record of swift and effective reaction to problems, one can expect economic rejuvenation at some point, accompanied by social and cultural exuberance. But will this mean returning to business-as-usual? And will the deep structures shaped by authoritarian politics and market fundamentalism continue to worsen income inequality, poverty, an over-dependency on exploited migrant workers, the neglect of heterotopic spaces of otherness, and a dogmatic refusal by the government to engage more widely and in good faith with a broader range of people and perspectives outside its circle?

Keywords Migrant worker dormitories · KTV lounges · COVID endemic · Neoliberal globalization · Political repression · Authoritarian populism · Political decadence

The chapters in this book have focused on Singapore's first year of living with COVID-19. The island-nation's overall reputation for dealing with the pandemic has so far been impressive. Even with one of the most open and therefore vulnerable economies in the world, the global city has been able to test, trace, isolate, treat, and vaccinate so effectively that its COVID death rate is among the lowest anywhere ("Coronavirus: Singapore confirms 34th casualty", 2021).

Singapore is named as one of the best places to live in during the pandemic (Hong, 2021). Its government has already charted a roadmap to normalcy, anticipating a shift from pandemic to endemic, when living with COVID-19 will feel like living with the common flu (Tham, 2021). And the Singapore government will no doubt draw practical lessons from the experience so that it can prepare the country for future pandemics, just as it did when SARS hit in 2003 (Shanmugaratnam, 2021).

However, Singapore's record has been far from perfect. Within the first year, as several chapters in this book have analysed from different angles, there was an outbreak in migrant worker dormitories that, at its peak in April 2020, numbered more than 1,000 new cases every day. Migrant workers make up 90% of all people in Singapore who have tested positive.

Most of them are Bangladeshi workers, who continue today to be housed in large, highly profitable, and privately run gated dormitories located on the margins of the island, segregated from local people. Typically overcrowded, poorly ventilated, and unsanitary, their rooms can accommodate up to 20 workers, making it nearly impossible still to practice strict social distancing. It has not been entirely clear whether dormitory operators failed to comply with government regulations, or whether regulations were too ambiguous in detailing standards and assigning responsibilities, or whether the enforcement of these regulations was just too lax. It was very likely a combination of these factors, skewed by a general inclination of the neoliberal state to act in favour of big businesses.

Over several months, the dormitories were placed under a strict lockdown, which only loosened as the infection numbers came under control. Today, their movements very much restricted, these migrant workers grapple with mental health and suicide, feeling like prisoners in their dormitories, uncertain about their own futures, and the well-being of their families back home ("Singapore's migrant workers", 2021).

To many, it might seem like the dormitory clusters—although certainly a serious matter—were just a blemish in an otherwise stellar record of successful crisis management by a high-capacity government responsible for developing Singapore from a "Third World" to a "First World" country in a very short period. Made up of very capable technocrats with a pragmatic outlook, this government focused on results, were quick to react to problems as they surfaced, and never took its eye away from the unsentimental task of keeping its globally embedded economy going as a vital part of national survival.

Some might argue that no government is perfect, not even this one, and that the authorities and countless other people in Singapore who volunteered their support did the best they could, in the context of an unprecedented and unpredictable pandemic of this scale and magnitude. The chapters in this book have not disagreed with this position. However, they have attempted to explain the dormitory clusters and other lapses as symptoms of deeper structural problems. This is important to do as it can provide insight into whether these kinds of problems will manifest again and again in occasional eruptions and disruptions, which are painful but manageable. Or whether they will lead to more systemically destructive outcomes over time, which will either ruin Singapore eventually or create the opportunity to rebuild something better.

From Dormitories to Lounges

In 2021, in Singapore's second year of living with the COVID-19 pandemic, there were serious virus outbreaks in the local community just as the government confidently laid out its roadmap for returning to normalcy amid low infection rates. The most serious was the cluster at KTV lounges, possibly linked to a growing number of other clusters, including a very concerning one in a fishery port.

Since October 2020, in response to industry pressures, the government allowed nightclub venues to continue operations, but only as food and beverage establishments. Not surprisingly, several of them breached safe management measures. Many also continued illegally to operate as karaoke lounges, where "butterfly" hostesses mostly in Singapore on social visit passes flitted from patron to patron, and sometimes from lounge to lounge, offering services of a sexual nature (Amierul, 2021). In these circumstances, the virus could spread easily and fast. And it did, forming rapidly spreading clusters that stymied the government's plan to return Singapore to a state of normalcy. The government started to clamp down on these illegal businesses, while heightening restrictions on the public, limiting their social group size to two and completely disallowing dining-in at all food and beverage establishments.

The government's swift action was admirable, but reactive instead of proactive. In the first place, how could such a serious lapse have occurred in a country like Singapore, which has the advantage of size, a high-capacity government, and a generally compliant citizenry.

Singapore's pragmatic approach to the sex trade might offer some insight. The government takes a realist position on prostitution, which, though officially illegal, it believes can never be eliminated. To prevent it from simply disappearing underground, as it did in Singapore's colonial past when prohibition was attempted, the government takes a pragmatic approach, containing and regulating it in designated red-light areas such as Geylang, which is also where some of the best local food may be found. Brothels are allowed to operate in these areas if they comply with standards and if registered sex workers receive regular medical check-ups. Outside these designated areas, there are also several places where sex work seems to be tolerated. However, the line becomes increasingly blurred. Some KTV lounges serve as fronts for illegal brothels in this ambiguous space, where behaviour is slippery and enforcement light.

As Andrea Dugo argued in his chapter, "even issues of public morality are put through the pragmatic-neoliberal sieve". Like the casinos that were allowed to be built in Singapore once the government was convinced that the economic benefits would outweigh the social costs, red-light areas in Singapore have for decades been a realist-pragmatic approach that not only accepted the inevitability of the sex trade and its role in maintaining stability in a high-stress and often emasculating society, but also acknowledged the broader commercial value that such work contributed to the larger economy. In general, this approach assumes that certain things like gambling and paying for sex—harmful though they may be—can never be eliminated, that they should be allowed if the economic benefits are clear, and that efforts should be made to minimize the social costs, including providing care and assistance to the casualties.

This would explain why the authorities could be persuaded to allow the nightclubs to continue operating, even though strict adherence to the "only F&B" stipulation would have been hard to imagine outside of the most naïve circles. And the authorities were certainly not naïve. It is therefore difficult to explain why they would have taken such a risk without ensuring the highest levels of surveillance and that the agencies assigned to enforce the new rules were capable of doing so. Family-friendly KTVs, restaurants, bars, and hawker stalls that complied with regulations had to pay the price for the errant behaviour of unscrupulous nightclub operators and their recalcitrant customers. These legitimate and mostly small businesses, which had already endured enormous losses and had been subjected to very frequent checks by an army of government-appointed safe distancing "ambassadors" and "enforcement officers", faced severe financial difficulty and many more were expected to close for good. Singaporeans, already worn down by one-and-a-half years of COVID-19 and looking forward to some semblance of normalcy, were furious.

While some of this fury was directed, moral panic style, towards foreign women who were illegally providing these sexual services as hostesses, most directed their outrage at the errant operators of these shady lounges. Geylang, other red-light areas, and the ambiguous spaces of KTV lounges that provide sexual services have been treated as a heterotopia, a space of otherness, but also one whose spatial boundaries have been sharpened by moral boundaries. In outwardly conservative Singapore, where prostitution is illegal but tolerated, foreign female sex workers, the businesspeople who employed them, and the wealthy men who patronized them,were easily stigmatized, drawing critical attention away from the authorities, who took great care to rebut accusations of culpability and to discredit critics (Lim, 2021a, b).

Hongwu Lyu and Aymeric Vo Quang, in their chapter, discussed how stigmatization and the moral panic that is often associated with it have historically weakened public health efforts to control such disease outbreaks as tuberculosis, HIV/AIDS, and even SARS in Singapore. In the case of COVID-19, South Asian migrant workers were not only stigmatized as culturally backward and unhygienic bearers of the disease, but also segregated from the local community through spaces of exclusion within "clean and green" Singapore. The money-making dormitories capitalized on the stigmatization of foreigners whom many Singaporeans grudgingly accepted into their country to provide low-waged labour that the neoliberal global city depended on, like a drug, to keep cost of living and doing business low. The hypocrisy of desiring and at the same time despising low-waged labour and sex work produced the two heterotopias of migrant worker dormitories (as Carolin Bernhard and Mara Ellemunt argued in their chapter) and red-light areas, spaces of otherness that neoliberal globalization feeds off and makes invisible to the beneficiaries of capitalism in its most morally indiscriminate form.

The relative neglect of these spaces reflected in their ineffective regulation makes them policy blind spots, in which the unexpected can expectedly emerge. The serious COVID-19 clusters have demonstrated this dramatically. Independent civil society organizations that advocate for migrant worker interests have warned the authorities of the dangers to which they seemed insufficiently attentive. However, the elitist state finds it difficult to engage productively and respectfully with those outside its tent, treating independent civil society activists not only as undesirable troublemakers, but often as opponents to be crushed.

FROM PANDEMIC TO ENDEMIC

Singapore was among the first in the world to announce a roadmap for returning to normalcy, when COVID-19 transforms from pandemic to endemic and comes to resemble the flu. It planned to loosen restrictions in stages once enough people had been vaccinated and there was certainty that its hospitals had adequate capacity to treat those who did get infected. Some safe management measures would continue to be required in public. There would be tweaks to the system, mainly the establishment of new institutional capacities for dealing with future pandemics.

Given Singapore's track record of swift and effective reaction to problems, as Johanna Dirlewanger-Lücke and Junhao Li described in their chapter, one can expect economic rejuvenation at some point, accompanied by social and cultural exuberance, just from the sheer joy that freedom brings. But will this mean returning to business-as-usual? And will the deep structures shaped by authoritarian politics and market fundamentalism continue to worsen income inequality, poverty, an overdependency on exploited migrant workers, the neglect of heterotopic spaces of otherness, and a dogmatic refusal by the government to engage more widely and in good faith with a broader range of people and perspectives outside its establishment circle?

Johanna Dirlewanger-Lücke and Junhao Li doubt that the government will be willing and able to change very much even in the face of electoral pressures to do so. Davide Brugola and Michael Flood doubt that the government will change course from its unsustainable immigration policies that have created an overdependency on cheap migrant labour without a commensurate sense of responsibility for their wellbeing. While Hongwu Lyu and Aymeric Vo Quang caution against social stigmatization and moral panic in implementing public health measures, Carolin Bernhard and Mara Ellemunt are doubtful that systemic change will happen as the government's mindset will continue to be shackled by notions of spatial scarcity, profit maximization, and the segregation of migrant otherness as core principles driving its technical solutions. Andrea Dugo urges the government to beef up its system of social protection so that Singapore can be ready for a reformed neoliberal globalization that adapts to survive the COVID-19 pandemic.

A New Authoritarianism

COVID-19 revealed both strengths and weaknesses in the Singapore system, over which the PAP has prevailed since 1959. The survivalist instincts of a post-independence generation continue into the present in the form of a collective determination to keep nation-state and global-city Singapore safe, peaceful, and prosperous, in the common belief that Singapore's success, no matter how impressive, is always fragile. For decades, the Singapore government has enjoyed uncommonly high levels of popular trust, legitimizing its paternalism and authoritarian methods well beyond what any electoral process can achieve. This trust has been built upon a stellar historical record of governmental achievement, which earlier generations of Singaporeans had experienced as rapid and substantial material advancement in their own lives.

Thus, when COVID-19 struck, the government could count on a large stock of social capital. Singaporeans generally abided by the restrictions placed on their behaviour in daily life, for some an inconvenience, for many others a terrible hardship. But Singaporeans grit their teeth, empathized, and did whatever they could to help those among them who were most in need, including the most vulnerable foreigners.

The second instinct, which this book has described in terms of neoliberal globalization, was honed since the late 1980s. This market-fundamentalist instinct meant that Singapore's public sector always kept an eye on efficiency and cost-savings, storing up enormous national reserves that could be drawn upon in times of need. COVID-19 was such an occasion. And the government was able to roll out generous support measures, particularly aimed at employers and businesses, in the expectation that others down the economic and social hierarchy would be helped by the trickling down of benefits.

But it was this same neoliberal instinct that held back when it came to state welfare provision. Thus, as global-city Singapore became increasingly entrenched in economic globalization and technological development radically transformed the economy and nature of work, the tightly managed welfare system did not do enough to redistribute from globalization's winners to its losers. Inequality of income and wealth became more pronounced, not only at the abstract statistical level, but also at the level of lived experience, intersecting with other dimensions of inequality along the lines of race, language, religion, gender, sexuality, age, and nationality. Meritocracy was rapidly rigidifying into elitism, slowing down social mobility, focusing on reward, but still insisting upon the individualization of success and failure in a Darwinian celebration of hyper-competition. More and more Singaporeans felt left behind and disrespected in one of the wealthiest countries in the world. Meanwhile, the technocratic elite seemed unsympathetic, at times arrogant and bullying in its manner, style, and insensitive choice of words. The top looked down with condescension, horror, and even disgust, while the bottom looked up with resentment, cynicism, and even envy.

These neoliberal-globalist conditions have created fertile ground for the germination of the third instinct, which relates to what this book has described as authoritarian populism. The experience of relative deprivation augmented by feelings of resentment, cynicism, and envy, and the hardship brought on by the COVID-19 pandemic all converge to unearth latent racist attitudes hitherto repressed beneath ideological layers of multiracial harmony. When repressed racism returns, it intersects with xenophobic tendencies, where the threat to the Singapore that locals used to know is projected onto the figure of the foreigner. Moral panic is the usual expression of these growing concerns. Both elite and working-class foreigners are susceptible to being singled out as folk devils. Meanwhile, the technocratic neoliberal elite, who are seen as responsible for pro-foreigner policies, are also viewed with increasing hostility, quickly depleting decades of accumulated trust in political leadership and public institutions.

However, this technocratic elite's pro-foreigner policies are by no means uniform. In the context of a bifurcated flow of immigrants in Singapore, every effort is made to attract global talent and wealthy foreigners to live and work in Singapore and perhaps eventually become citizens. Many Singaporeans have been conditioned to view such an approach as necessary for the nation's survival and success, but they increasingly question whether the best talents are in fact coming to Singapore, whether locals are being displaced by foreigners where good jobs are concerned, and whether the government's liberal immigration policies are proportionate and sufficiently discriminating. With COVID-19, the competition for jobs has become an especially fraught political issue. The image of experienced and well-qualified middle-class Singaporeans losing their jobs and turning to precarious work in the gig economy is finding a worrisome place in the public imagination.

With working-class migrants, other than surveillance in public spaces, the government's approach has been "light touch". In the cynical perspective of neoliberal globalization, migrant workers are merely labour input that businesses require and pro-business governments should make available—the cheaper, less protected, and more dispensable the better. Even housing them as far away as possible from the mainstream society has become a very profitable enterprise. It is in that context, then, that the dormitory outbreaks and the continued restrictions on the human rights of locked-down dormitory residents can be so readily understood.

Although the PAP government's first-year record of dealing with the pandemic is mixed, the longer the path to endemicity, the more frustrated people will be with the government as more mistakes will be committed and compounded, and the people's patience and goodwill will run dry. Acutely aware of the political risks and what this could mean for the thus-far lacklustre succession to the 4G leadership, the technocratic elite has sharpened their instruments of political repression and are resorting to the politics of fear. In addition to the law against online misinformation (Protection from Online Falsehoods and Manipulation Act, POFMA) that commenced in October 2019 is a new even more draconian law, the Foreign Interference (Countermeasures) Act (FICA), passed swiftly with minimal parliamentary debate in October 2021 to counter foreign interference. The PAP government's political opponents have been especially concerned about being targeted and neutered by these laws. In fact, anyone who values a diversity of perspectives and views as requisite conditions for resilience in governance will be concerned about the chill factor from such a high- and heavy-handed approach to the "truth" and its brute power to silence alternative voices. Indeed, the record shows that POFMA has mainly been used against the PAP's opponents, especially during the general elections of 2020 (Aravindan, 2019).

So now, the government expresses at least three different views of foreigners: those whom it likes and wants to attract for high-quality economic value and potential citizenship (foreign talent), those who are useful to business interests but must be kept cheap and dispensable (migrant workers), and those who are demonized for getting involved in Singapore's domestic affairs (foreign originators of hostile information campaigns). In the case of foreign talent and migrant workers, the government actively defends its neoliberal-globalist position, augmenting the claims with sometimes hysterical assertions of national survival. In the case of foreign interference, it drums up nativist-populist support against foreigners, in similar ways as when it condemned theories and concepts critical of the system as "Western" ideas that have no authentic and rightful place in Singapore. Such ideas have included "human rights', "liberal democracy", and "critical race theory". This performance of post-colonial criticality has the power to muster populist support for essentially neoliberal policies. Elsewhere, I develop the notion of "neoliberal populism" to characterize this political fluidity, arguing that it is dangerous politics and a clear sign of political decadence.

Singapore may once have had pragmatic leadership willing and able to make bold and far-sighted policies. But ironically, the success of that heroic generation has been bequeathed to the next as success formulas, hardened into dogma, yet modulated by the seductive notes of neoliberal globalization that narrow judgement and moral reasoning to the simple logic of the market, tuned to efficiency and growth. As the COVID-19 pandemic has demonstrated, this political hardness turns out to be brittle in the face of the challenges of an increasingly volatile, uncertain, complex, and ambiguous world. Playing with authoritarian-populist forces to secure a neoliberal-globalist agenda is a decadent kind of politics that signals deadlock, stagnation, exhaustion, decay, and ultimately decline.

References

Amierul Rashid (2021) "'There are quite many SIA girls in KTVs': Singapore hostess spills the beans on ins and outs of industry", *AsiaOne*, 30 July.

Aravindan, Aradhana (2019) "Singapore 'fake news' law ensnares government critics", *Reuters*, 16 October.

"Coronavirus: Singapore confirms 34th casualty, surpassing Sars death toll; South Korea eyes Asia travel bubbles" (2021) *South China Morning Post*, 9 June.

Hong, Jinshan (2021) "Singapore is now the world's best place to be during COVID", *Bloomberg*, 27 April.

Lim, Min Zhang (2021a) "Nikkei commentary on KTV outbreak 'full of inaccuracies': MHA official", *The Straits Times*, 29 July.

Lim, Min Zhang (2021b) "Shanmugam questions motives of writer behind 'fictional' Nikkei piece on KTV Covid-19 cluster", *The Straits Times*, 29 July.

Shanmugaratnam, Tharman (2021) "Learning from crisis", *Ethos*, Issue 11, June.

"Singapore's migrant workers have endured interminable lockdowns" (2021) *The Economist*, 19 June.

Tham, Yuen-C (2021) "Singapore preparing roadmap for living with Covid-19", *The Straits Times*, 24 June.

INDEX